Living is Risky

Living is Risky

✦

Staying Alive
in Spite of Ourselves

Felix M. Berardo
University of Florida

iUniverse, Inc.
New York Lincoln Shanghai

Living is Risky
Staying Alive in Spite of Ourselves

iUniverse books may be ordered through booksellers or by contacting:

iUniverse
2021 Pine Lake Road, Suite 100
Lincoln, NE 68512
www.iuniverse.com
1-800-Authors (1-800-288-4677)

ISBN-13: 978-0-595-40274-8 (pbk)
ISBN-13: 978-0-595-84648-1 (ebk)
ISBN-10: 0-595-40274-7 (pbk)
ISBN-10: 0-595-84648-3 (ebk)

Printed in the United States of America

This book is dedicated to my parents, Rocco and Maria Berardo, who took the risk of leaving their home in Italy to start a new life in this country. Immigrants, as is well known, face many obstacles in their efforts to assimilate, including ghettoization, prejudice, loneliness, and a host of uncertainties. But throughout my upbringing, they faced these difficulties, often in a hostile environment, and overcame them with courage and determination.

And to my wife, Dr. Donna H. Berardo, who faced a different kind of risk in deciding to marry me. I am not ashamed to say that she is the anchor in this marriage. Her adventurous spirit never ceases to astound me.

Contents

Acknowledgments

Most books, this one included, would never come to fruition without the encouragement and contributions of many significant others. I want, therefore, specifically to acknowledge them. Dr. Hernan Vera, whose ideas and editorial and computer expertise have been crucial. Dr. Donna H. Berardo, without whose encouragement, daily support and insights, contributed to the confidence one needs in writing a book. Dr. Constance Shehan, whom I have mentored for many years and who is delightfully now mentoring me. Her writing ability in particular has been treasured. Dr. Menno Vellinga and his wife, Kathy, whose reading of the manuscript has resulted in remarkable alterations of the text. Dr. Gordon Streib and Ruth Streib, who remain always available as consultants and a sounding board for what I have written. And of course, I acknowledge the many students who read the manuscript in its original form and made many significant suggestions. I am grateful for Steven Arxer's editorial help. In the end, I bear full responsibility for any errors, omissions, and the like.

Preface

This book has its beginnings in an earlier issue of <u>Death Studies</u>, a journal devoted to thanathological issues.[1] That particular issue was titled *Survivorship: the Other Side of Death and Dying*. Its contents fell within what I called **survivor education**. The concept of survivor education has, in fact, been a major component of a course I introduced many years ago at the University of Florida: The **Sociology of Death and Survivorship.** This work continues that emphasis on survival.

My professional career has been that of an academic sociologist, a person who teaches and conducts research within a university setting. Hence, most of my publications to date were written with that intellectual audience in mind. However, my goal from the beginning of this book has been to reach a larger audience—one that would reach beyond the community of scholars to an enlightened lay public. I wasn't quite sure how to define that larger audience. Fortunately, Melvin Konner did that for me in *Why The Reckless Survive…and Other Secrets of Human Nature:*

> Who is this general reader? Someone who loves to learn but does not want to feel quite like a pupil again. Someone who appreciates the subtleties of language but does not want to keep getting up to go to the dictionary. Someone who knows perfectly well that complex ideas can usually be expressed without gobbledygook. Someone who wants to feel that reading is conversation, not lecture or catechism.[2]

Hopefully, both the academic and curious general reader will find the present book interesting as well as informative.

To attract such a mixed audience requires a different style of communication, not normally employed by the university professor/scientist. I have found that this is not a simple task. It requires a conscious effort to overcome decades of habits of expression and replace them with a different mode of presentation, one relatively free of technical abstractions as well as arcane and elusive professional jargon. After many years of writing in this mode, one is reluctant to leave its habituated and comforting embrace.

I am not sure to what extent I have succeeded in making that linguistic transition. In due time, however, members of the targeted audience will let me know, one way or the other. The lay public, whom I hope will be attracted to the topics covered, will probably be quick to make up its mind. Professional colleagues, of course, will not hesitate to render ponderous pronouncements as to whether the time or money is worth the scholarship evidenced by this work. This I welcome. My skin is thick. Quite frankly, however, I would be more interested in the reaction of students. I say this because often as I worked on a section or chapter I would have them in mind as a relevant sector of the larger audience I seek. I have found over the years that they can, perhaps in different ways, be as perceptive and critical as any of my professional reference groups. Hence, I gird myself for their response as well.

While the reader will discern many useful hints about "how to stay alive in spite of ourselves" in the following pages, this is not a how-to-book, at least in the usual sense of that genre. The authors of many such books lead readers to believe that what is offered in the way of advice is based upon well-established scientific confirmations. All too often, however, the advice given is no more than the writer's personal intuition or view of the world, couched in his or her own peculiar brand of pop psychology or sociology, and catchy words or phrases along with overly simplistic solutions to complex problems. While many such books do contain some helpful information and counsel, the public would do well to approach their promises of a better tomorrow with some caution. The keys to a better life, unfortunately, do not come in simple-to-read and easy-to-follow prescriptions wrapped in well-packaged volumes right off the shelf of your local book store or in the latest issue of the voluminous so-called health magazines or newsletters that have proliferated across the land. While certain of these are clearly educational and informative, the outrageous promises offered by too many others often border on the ludicrous.

Advisory statements, to be sure, are by no means absent from the present book. Some specific guidelines, derived from scientifically based knowledge, as to how to avoid premature annihilation are inserted at various points throughout. However, I do not suffer from the illusion that most readers will immediately act on them. Why? Because they typically require a personal commitment to permanent changes in one's lifestyle. Most of us are either reluctant or unable to make such changes, especially if this means relinquishing the many pleasures gained from our current mode of living. Indeed, people seem averse to accepting advice or following it except, perhaps, when they *actively* seek it out *and* pay for it. As

Benjamin Franklin once observed, "we can give *advice*, but we cannot give *conduct*. Remember this: they that will not be counseled cannot be helped."

The disinclination to heed the voices of mature and seasoned others leads untold numbers of each generation to repeat the mistakes of their predecessors. A healthy skepticism is necessary in examining the latest pronouncements from "experts" about life choices and life paths. However, to dismiss blindly the accumulated wisdom of the past or the scientific evidence of the present regarding those ways of living which affect our health and welfare, can lead to unnecessary exposure to life-threatening conditions and sometimes unintended self-destruction. Change and adaptation are essential to survival. To live life to the fullest requires a purposeful shift away from attitudes which lead us to ignore the risks of our existence, toward a more rational model—one that takes advantage of the ever present potential for extending and enhancing the human condition. I believe the public is slowly but surely moving in that direction, and that bodes well for the future.

Readers may find the concept of vulnerability to be useful for understanding much of the material in this book. Although difficult to define precisely, vulnerability consists in the exposure to a risk without the resources adequate to cope with it. Vulnerability can occur at several levels. At the individual level, people engaging in risky behavior make themselves vulnerable to a variety of negative outcomes. For example, individuals who climb mountains without anything but their bare hands are placing themselves in danger. At the societal level hazards are imposed by events that place individuals at risk; for example, a pesticide that impacts the eco-system can render people vulnerable to a variety of hazards and irreversible outcomes. Finally, people can suffer from multiple vulnerabilities, such those in poverty who are discriminated racially, cannot afford health insurance, and who live in toxic or violent environments.[3]

Introduction

In the forest hills of Oregon, a middle-aged man sits in an underground bunker surrounded by canned and powdered food supplies, bottled water, various weapons and ammunition, reserves of electrical battery and generator power. He has mined the perimeter surrounding his bunker with explosives which can be armed to protect it from assault by those who might come to steal away his "life support" system. The man in the bunker is termed by himself and others as a *survivalist*, one of an apparently large number of Americans who plans to live long beyond any revolutionary change in society resulting from war, foreign invasion, economic collapse, technological breakdown, natural disasters, pollution, or dramatic decreases in energy and fuel resources.

No one knows exactly how many such "doomsdayers" there are but it is generally agreed that they number in the tens of thousands. Many subscribe newsletters, take survivalist training courses, and some even construct especially equipped survival homes which may include, among other things, well stocked fallout shelters, radiation suits, extra gasoline and auto parts, and home-made weapons. Others purchase underground condominiums, fitted with blast proof doors, eight inches of reinforced concrete overhead, and supplies of food in the walls and ceilings.[4,5,6]

On the other side of the continent, there is a 65-year-old attorney retiring from one of the nations' most prestigious, high-powered law firms. His entire career has been characterized by risk-taking and extreme job stress, yet he retires a healthy man who foresees years of leisurely retirement living. He has numerous counterparts in other occupations, including a highly visible personality who recently retired as head of one of the nation's leading automobile companies. Over the years, he has led that company through a series of crises and recoveries. These men represent a different kind of survivor. They are members of our rapidly growing older population, reflecting one segment of the so-called graying of America. They want to remain in good health, avoid risks, and live as long as possible in order to enjoy the fruits of their labor.

In Los Angeles, California, a much younger couple begin their four-times-a-day regimen of megadoses of vitamins, drugs and nutrients in a long term experiment they believe will result in prolonged life.[7,8] Their ideas are based upon the *free-radical hypothesis* of aging, which holds that highly reactive compounds, formed during metabolism attack and damage vital cell structures and thereby age the body. This deterioration process can be forestalled, they argue, by taking *antioxidants*, substances (mostly vitamins) that presumably prevent some of the damage caused by free radicals. They believe that they have probably increased their life expectancy by at least one year for each year they have followed the regimen. This is noteworthy, since the central premise of their work—that human life can be extended with mega doses of nutrients—lacks essential scientific confirmation. Nevertheless, they remain faithfully committed to their regimen. They want to look and feel young as long as possible, and to live a long and healthy life.

Meanwhile, the public has chosen not to await the arrival of definitive results regarding this matter. Despite the lack of conclusive evidence that vitamin supplements prevent serious illness, a growing proportion of the lay citizenry are consuming them in ever-increasing amounts. They apparently have come to perceive vitamins as possible preventives for heart disease, cancer, and many other disorders. In recent years sales of vitamins A, C, E, and beta carotene, in particular, have risen significantly. Companies have kept busy developing and marketing a range of antioxidant supplements, promoting their presumed radical-shielding ability, which supposedly helps ward off illness and disease.[9]

Many professionals are also ingesting daily doses of vitamins in the belief that antioxidants lower the risk of various diseases by blocking the action of highly reactive oxygen-containing chemicals—those free radicals. They are part of a *life-extension movement* that proliferates across the country in numerous seminars, institutes, and clinics. Participants are largely health conscious, high-income young professionals, the so-called "yuppies" (and more recently "grumpies"—Grown-Up Mature Professionals) who seek to retard the aging process and keep themselves immune from illnesses through dietary manipulation, exercise, and a variety of risk-avoidance strategies.[10] They pay little heed to warnings that many programs, products, and services that hold out the promise of retarding aging have very limited scientific basis or none at all. Nor are they deterred by evidence that "many popular life-extension pills are useless, dangerous, or both."[11] They too, want to retain their youthful appearance, remain healthy, and live as long as they possibly can.

Across the country and around the world, ethicists and many others debate whether we can decide for someone else that life isn't always preferable to death. The elderly have become the focus of this debate that has spawned several related questions. Can we put a price tag on life without devaluing it? Are the very old worth the cost of their heath care? Should life be judged solely by its "quality?"

Some have proposed that all medical care and treatment should be denied the elderly when they reach the end of their "natural life span," which they presume to be somewhere around or even before 80 years of age, so that our limited medical resources can be directed toward the younger generation.[12] Others have challenged such age-based rationing of health services, criticizing them from a variety of legal, economic, philosophical, medical, moral, and religious perspectives.[13] Their position is that people should be allowed to live as long as is possible under the circumstances, and that every effort should be made to preserve the quality of their existence.

Still other scientists are debating the value of ***caloric restriction*** as a means of achieving a healthier and longer life. Research has shown that laboratory mice subjected to such a regimen exhibit lower incidences of illness and infirmities, and extended life spans. Experiments are also underway to discover whether restricted diets can also work in primates. A major advocate of the calorie-cutting or weight loss approach argues that it will also work in humans, and has the potential for increasing our life span to about 140 years.[14] Others disagree. Some contend we may already be close to the maximum life span determined through evolution. Still others point out that the low-calorie life-extension findings contradict other research in nutrition and health. Noting that humans naturally tend to gain pounds as they grow older, that research indicates that in middle age or beyond, people with higher weights have a survival advantage, that is, they have lower death rates. Such findings, in turn, run contrary to other results that link being overweight to heart disease, diabetes, and high blood pressure.

Hence, the controversy over which approach to improving human aging and life extension continues unabated. Meanwhile, a variety of approaches to extend human longevity are being pursued, including ***cryonic preservation***, the freezing of a dead body until future advances in medicine can be brought to bear to revive the person and repair what killed them; ***transplantation***, involving continuous replacement of failed organs, with the potential for the entire body to be composed of new parts; ***prosthetic*** and ***cyborgs***, comprised of machine-human combinations (shades of the bionic man or woman); *identity reconstruction*, via cloning processes; and ***regeneration***, whereby repressed genes are activated to trigger cell tissue renewal.[15]

All these examples point toward a major focus of this book, namely, the area of survivorship. Webster's New Collegiate Dictionary defines this simply as "the state of being a survivor," and the latter as someone who continues "to exist or live after." One writer simply defines survival as "the desire to live." These are not very helpful definitions. They connote little of the life-enhancing, life-sustaining, and life-preserving subject matter we will be dealing with. In this book the terms survivor and survivorship are used in a much broader and inclusive sense to encompass a variety of states of existence and modes of action and reaction which directly and indirectly bear upon the length and quality of life. In this context, life-diminishing and life-threatening attitudes, behaviors, and conditions are included and made explicit, with a particular emphasis on risk-taking and risk-aversion.

At the most general level the contents of this volume are embraced by that long-standing question: why are some people healthy and others not? That important question, it has been noted, "has generated a vast academic literature, spanning many disciplines and many decades."[16] A completed and satisfactory response to that broad question has by no means been achieved by interested specialists from various scientific disciplines. Many of the "anomalous findings" derived from research directed at such an inquiry have yet to be resolved. There is, nevertheless, a growing body of accumulated evidence that identifies some of the major factors associated with continued good health over the life-cycle. This book examines some of that evidence and adds to it, by focusing more specifically on related and equally important questions such as: What allows some people to survive while others die in the same situation? What, if any, significant differences exist between those people who overcome a life-threatening illness and those who do not? Are some people more vulnerable than others to life events? What role does attitude play? For some, like this Episcopal priest, the answer is clear:

> Surviving involves attitude. A survivor refuses to give up, clings to a strong sense of hope, believes that life continues to hold deep meaning. A survivor remains open to positive alternatives, fresh options, new prospects for the future...A survivor honors life, supports it, goes on loving and offering unconditional love, and goes on living fully despite discouragements and setbacks...Stay open to new possibilities. Preserve a healthy attitude. Never lose hope.[17]

Do those who live the longest possess a particular set of social, psychological, or genetic attributes which set them apart from others? Is risk-taking related to longevity? How do habits and attitudes influence the probabilities of an early demise? Are certain personalities more prone to shorter lives? Is there a connection between mental and physical health? What role do interpersonal relationships play in extending the length of life? How do societal and global conditions promote or inhibit our ability to remain healthy survivors? What strategies can individuals implement to enhance the quality of their existence and to improve their life chances?

This book aims in part to provide a counterbalance to the voluminous literature on death and dying. In recent decades that literature has ballooned to the point where it is no longer possible to claim, as writers in the past legitimately could, that death is a taboo topic in American society. Indeed, by the end of the 1970s there already was far more written and published about death than anyone could possibly read or keep up with.[18] The rapid proliferation of death and dying classes in our high schools, colleges and universities, and the emergence of several specialty journals and professional organizations devoted to *Thanatology*—the study of death—further attest to the contemporary widespread interest in death education. What has been missing until relatively recently-and what this volume seeks to address—is the other side of death and dying, namely, **survivor education**[19] In more general terms it asks: "What are some of the major social factors that enhance life expectancy and the human condition?"

Such a focus is paramount for understanding why and how some people can increase life expectancy relative to their particular circumstances. Promoting life chances, of course, goes far beyond the maintenance of physical health. Survival strategies directly impinge on the *quality* of life as well—a quality that affects the social and psychological well-being of the individual with concomitant positive results for society. For example, many beneficial consequences would accrue from a significant reduction of the staggering financial costs that society currently bears for preventable illness, injury, disability, and premature death.

These financial consequences are extensive in scope. Coronary heart disease, for example, results in millions of deaths annually. This alone cost the nation approximately billions in direct and indirect costs. Add to this the victims of the other leading causes of premature death among adults (malignant neoplasm, cirrhosis of the liver, accidents, influenza and pneumonia, motor vehicle accidents, suicide and homicide) and the financial costs mount to increasingly staggering levels. Three decades ago the share of the Gross National Product going to medical services was 5 percent. It reached 12 percent in 1990, passed the 14 percent mark a few years later, is now 18 percent. However, lost economic productivity attendant to illness and early death compounds the impact of this problem. When these are factored in, then total costs of illness are even greater. Embedded in these costs are the associated monumental equivalents in pain and suffering. Much of this could be diminished or avoided through alterations in habits and attitudes that would enhance our lives and prevent premature death.

In the following pages I embrace both the individual and societal (including the medical and corporate) contexts that significantly influence our life potential. These contexts often overlap and interact as determinants of our health status. Scientists have increasingly come to acknowledge *antecedent social and behavioral risk factors* as "precursors of the biological processes by which disease becomes manifest."[20] Illustrative here would be tobacco use, alcohol and substance abuse, speeding and motor vehicle accidents, and socioeconomic status, including education, occupation, and income—all of which significantly influence the probabilities of sickness and premature death. This perspective is succinctly expressed by one analyst who notes: that two-thirds of all disease and premature death is due to behavioral and societal characteristics and is, therefore, theoretically avoidable. Negative health behaviors, rather than arising by chance reflect the social circumstances surrounding a person's life…The fundamental characteristics of a society determine the behaviors of its members, and these behaviors are the major determinants of health.[21]

This perspective implicitly speaks to the controversy that arose during the early 1990s in the United States over a proposed national health care system. One assumption underlying such a system, and associated policies, is that if unimpeded access to such a system is provided, people will reap the benefits of improved health and longevity, and the nation's health bill will thereby be reduced. That assumption may be questionable, given the risks that people take and the alternative pathways to daily living that many choose to follow. Many of those pathways reflect sociocultural influences (example, cigarette smoking) and eventually lead to disease, illness, and even early death. With this perspective in mind, the initial chapters examine the implications of personal habits, attitudes, and lifestyles for human survival. Individual lifestyles bear directly on the length and quality of our existence on this earth. Certain habits and attitudes which reflect these personal styles are examined in terms of their life-endangering potential. Particular attention is given to how several important cultural and personal attitudes affect life chances and one's ability to live fully according to one's given potential. The emphasis on longevity does not mean I favor it over the quality of life. The fullness of life, most would agree, is not related to years alone but also to the caliber of our existence.

Separate chapters are devoted to how individuals cope with stress. The link between stress and survivorship is receiving prominent attention in medical and psychosocial research. The dynamics of this linkage are not fully understood. However, it is known that stress, if not properly dealt with, can have severe pathological consequences on one's immune, cardiovascular, and central nervous systems. These consequences can be deadly. There are a variety of practical procedures one can use to minimize the negative repercussions of stress, thereby increasing one's chances for living.

Subsequent chapters focus on the influence that a person's social networks have on the life span. Here we will examine the connections between social ties, health status, and death. There is strong evidence that social relationships and networks are life-enhancing and contribute to longevity. The *broken heart syndrome* illustrates the increased mortality risk that follows the loss of a spouse and subsequent emotional and physiological consequences of severe grief. Factors associated with the higher mortality rates of males are scrutinized. It appears that for men, remarriage may have life-extension potentials. Enduring human relationships, especially with significant others, seem to prevent illness and premature death, although we are not entirely sure why. Nevertheless, a lifelong effort to establish and maintain a network of continuous intimate social ties apparently helps preserve life.

Eventually we shift to the societal level, where mortality differentials are examined in terms of demographic and regional characteristics, as well as in the context of world wide social change. Here the focus is on the societal context, on factors that influence life chances. Observations have been made of strong linkages between patterns of mortality and where one lives and works, as well as how these patterns vary by socioeconomic status and race. The notion that your location in the social strata can constrain or expand your ability to pursue healthy living is well documented. Most people are generally aware that technological innovations can and do affect patterns of living. Hence, the question of how major changes in technology and related mores of American society have impacted our survival potential is also taken up. In addition, a number of significant patterns of behavior that diminish the length and quality of life are discussed. They range from individual activities (for example, smoking, alcohol, or drug abuse) to national policies influencing family planning and the control of toxic agents. The threat to human survival posed by overpopulation and environmental contamination on the societal and global level is particularly pertinent in this age of large-scale technological innovations, and hence is examined in some detail.

A major and prominent theme throughout this volume is the role of risks and risk-taking in relation to survival. Risk factors are among the core categories of variables employed in epidemiologic studies because they are seen as being associated with or explaining particular health outcomes.[22] As we shall see, these are complex concepts and, as many scientists have discovered, not susceptible to simple definitions. For example, the term *risk factor* not only "embraces both direct causes or disease agents, but it also covers personal characteristics that make individuals more or less prone to a particular disease or injury."[23] Nevertheless, an awareness of the many unnecessary hazards individuals voluntarily expose themselves to, as well as an understanding of the risks to our lives imposed by others, is essential to our survival. For this reason, we early on explore the question of why people engage in unnecessary, life-threatening ventures. It is a difficult question and a variety of possible answers has been offered by professionals engaged in the emerging discipline of risk analysis. One of the more intriguing questions is: "Why would an intelligent, well-informed person, with easy access to and understanding of the latest knowledge, disregard that information and continue to place his or her life in jeopardy?" Or as one student of the psychology of excitement put it, why would an otherwise rational person choose to cross over to "the dangerous edge" of experience and place themselves at risk, or continue "playing with fire" in situations where potentially dire consequences are obvious?"[24] Why anyone considering behavior with life-threatening implications would weigh the risks and consequences, and elect to choose the risks? We all know such people. In fact, we may be one of them.

Death educators generally agree with the principle that true maturity is achieved only when we have learned to face the reality of our own death and then shaped our ways of living accordingly.[25] Implicit here is the notion that to die well one must first develop a *rational* form of living, that is, one must be an educated survivor. Death education and survivor education, therefore, are complementary sides of the same coin. A primary objective of the former is to assist people in coming to grips with their feelings and attitudes toward death and the dying process. A major goal of the latter is to sensitize people to those attitudes, behaviors, and conditions that imperil their life paths and decrease their longevity. Death education and survivor education presume that through knowledge and the achievement of these goals, death will become less fearful and life will be more rewarding and enjoyable.[26]

The ability to maximize life expectancy through a rational form of living is a function of personal choices *and* societal incentives. Within either context strategies can be implemented to reduce mortality and morbidity risks at the same time that they strengthen our survival capability.[27] These strategies involve an *active orientation*—the person consciously examines and then pursues behavioral options designed to minimize risks and achieve a longer and healthier life. Such activity is both preventive and promotive; one avoids smoking to prevent lung and heart disease; one walks or jogs to promote the utility of these same respiratory and circulatory systems. These more obvious strategies, along with a host of more subtle but equally important tactics, comprise those elements of death education that contribute to the art of living. Our major emphasis then, is not so much on death and dying as on the human potential for living. The objective is to remain alive *and* healthy for as long as possible—in spite of ourselves.

1

The Risk Factor: The Role of Attitudes and Habits

It has been suggested that the best hope for achieving a longer and healthier life lies in voluntary efforts derived from personal choices.[28] This means that individual change must be directed toward the modification of lifestyles and the choices associated with them. Every lifestyle is a complex of related attitudes, habits, and other behaviors that, in essence, constitute a *deathstyle*.[29] Each deathstyle in turn carries with it various degrees of risk-taking.

Our survival potential both in terms of quality and longevity is significantly enhanced or diminished by certain attitudes and habits and their associated risks. This dimension of survivor education is the central focus of this chapter. While it largely concentrates on individual culpability, the societal context is not ignored. Indeed, as we will note in later chapters, threats to our welfare often come from institutional or corporate activities that are beyond individual control. An over-emphasis on individual responsibility has the potential for denying broader social responsibilities for health and disease. Moreover, it is recognized that there are limits to the ability of individuals to constantly and completely exert self-control over their own health. As one critic warned, strict advocacy of a philosophy of self-control often carrys with it "a large dose of asceticism."[30] Few of us are willing or able to practice extreme self-denial, which can sometimes lead to abstention from the normal pleasures of life. It is important to keep in mind, therefore, that many life-threatening conditions are also externally imposed as, for example, industrial air pollution. Hence, an adequate understanding of who is at risk, how people incur risk, and why they remain at risk must ultimately derive from looking at the relationships between social and cultural contexts, including powerful economic forces, and individual psychological motivations to engage in or disengage from risk behaviors. The assumption and perpetuation of the cigarette smoking habit, is a good example of such relationships.[31]

When Is A Risk A Risk?

Major difficulties arise in both the definition and perception of risk. Some people, although appearing to others to be engaging in dangerous and death-defying activity, do not consider themselves as takers of risks. For example, while gathering material for a book on why people take risks, Ralph Keyes interviewed Philippe Petit, a tightrope walker well known for traversing a cable stretched between the twin towers of the New York World Trade Center, and similar feats. To his surprise, Petit repeatedly insisted that he did not view his wire walking as risk-taking.[32] The amount of preparation for and control over his activity apparently minimized, at least in his mind, the element of chance, and hence his fear of danger.

In interviews with many other people Keyes, like other students of this subject, soon encountered a wide range of meanings associated with the idea of risk. Coming up with a useful definition became a major challenge. He soon discovered that different people define danger differently. What may be perceived as a risk by one individual may not be perceived as such by another. In other words, the definition of risk is relative.

> most of us are far more conscious of the risks we're avoiding than those we're taking. This is why so few of us admit to being risk takers. And because we are so aware of the risks we avoid, it's easy to assume that others are taking bigger risks—especially if they're the ones we're ducking. Except they may be ducking risks we're taking. So risk, in this sense, is in the eye of the beholder. Or more precisely, in the fears of the beholder (p.21).

It is, of course, not all that simple. Keyes offers his own somewhat abstract definition of risk as "an act involving fear of possible loss." Again, in his words:

> Real fear of possible loss is central to actual risk. Objective danger counts less than perceived danger. Too many so-called risks are ones that the risk taker feels can't be lost no matter what the actual odds are. A pure risk taken with the full awareness of possible loss is rare. Most acts of apparent daring are usually motivated by a mishmash of ignorance, bravado, derring-do, carelessness, reduced stakes, peer pressure, and the desire to impress (p. 25).

The idea here is that we tend to define only those activities that would scare us as risky. Hence his question: "If you don't fear losing your life, is it a risk to play Russian roulette?" In short, our personal assessment of risk includes many other factors besides objective danger.

Many of the definitions found in the literature surrounding this topic are, unfortunately, either statistically complex[33] or vague, if not simplistic. My Random House Dictionary offers the following: "exposure to the chance of injury or loss; a hazard or dangerous chance." Is this sufficient to work with? Is this view of risk as the *probability* of some *adverse* effect or hazard a more precise offering?[34] It is likely, for instance, to ignore the often positive aspects of risk and uncertainty in people's lives. The development a working definition of risk, one that is easily subject to measurement, can be an arduous task, as many have discovered. However, our survival potential—both in terms of quality of living and life extension—is clearly enhanced or diminished by certain attitudes and habits and their associated risks.

That people vary widely in their perceptions of risk is evident. That there are different kinds of risks and different degrees of risk-taking is similarly self evident. Some risks are more acceptable than others. Moreover, as Imperato and Mitchell remind us, some risks are *chosen* while other are *imposed*.[35] In the case of chosen risks, it is assumed that an individual takes a specific action with some knowledge of the hazards he or she will be exposed to. Illustrative here are cigarette smoking, the non-use of safety belts in automobiles, and living in regions of the country notorious for hazardous mud slides or disastrous earthquakes. Any number of subtle and explicit factors can configure in a person's mind which allow them to perceive such risks as acceptable. "These factors interact in a decision making process both conscious and unconscious, resulting in what we perceive as our free choice" (p.9).

Imposed risks, on the other hand, are characterized by the belief that individuals have limited control over their exposure to a given hazard. The drug industry provides many examples of imposed risks. Perhaps one of the best known historical examples is *thalidomide*. In the early 1960s it was prescribed to many pregnant women to treat the nausea of morning sickness. Unfortunately, thalidomide invaded the developing fetus resulting in many of these mothers giving birth to deformed babies. Also illustrative here is *oralflex*, which was approved for marketing by the Federal Drug Administration and then sold to the public. It was subsequently discovered that Oralflex was actually dangerous to a segment of the population too small to be detected in testing, but large enough to warrant a recall.

Over the years such incidents have led to greater recognition that drugs ingested by pregnant women can seriously alter fetal development. The plight and suffering of so-called *cocaine babies* dramatically illustrate the potential damage and life-threatening implications of unnecessary fetal exposure to drugs.

The financial costs of treating such victims, of course, further exacerbate an already overburdened health care system.

Imposed risks also include many other hazards produced by new technologies but which the federal government cannot adequately test for safety. These potential hazards range from those associated with the irradiation of our daily food to those associated with a major nuclear accident. There are, in fact, so many hazards that the government could never adequately regulate them all. Even if this were possible, it would not necessarily resolve other problems related to imposed risks. For example, there is the dilemma of being forced to choose one type of threat over another, as in the debate over selecting coal or nuclear power sources of energy. Unfortunately, the solution to such dilemmas all too often advocated by elected officials is to play into the hands of representatives of industry by allowing them to get away with "propagandizing the public, influencing pubic policy, controlling the nature and flow of information, wearing down the regulatory agencies, minimizing the risks, and using diversionary tactics" (p.85). In this context, the imposed part of an imposed risk does not mean that it is unavoidable, but rather that others have selected one risk over another without consulting the individuals or communities who will be subjected to the hazard.

The main difference between these choice and imposition categories appears to be the level of control that a person may or may not have over a given risk. Numerous factors come into play in trying to assess the amount of control an individual will be able to exercise in any given situation. First, there are variable levels of information possessed by different people about the same hazard. Moreover, it is often presumed that giving people more and accurate information will lead them to reduce exposure to threats to their health and their lives. This is a dubious presumption. Despite massive education programs about lethal risks, large numbers of people do smoke, fail to buckle up their car seat belts, and so on. Second, there are also differing levels of actual *physical* control over exposure to perilous conditions. In such cases, no amount of information can provide protection because the danger is ubiquitous—such as worldwide air pollution. Despite difficulties of measurement, the admittedly broad distinctions between chosen and imposed risks furnish us with the beginnings of a more helpful definition and understanding of that concept.

Measuring Risks: A Brief Discourse

Some investigators have sought to develop specific indicators of the actual severity of one type of risk as opposed to another. If such designations were available or easy to calculate they might help us to compare more effectively competing threats to our well-being. It is difficult, for example, to assess accurately the relative risks between driving 2,000 miles across the country in an automobile and flying a similar distance in an airplane. Which activity has the greater life-threatening potential?

Two German physicians, Urquhart and Heilman, became interested in this problem of relative risk assessment and subsequently wrote a book on the subject.[36] In discussing various reasons underlying the public's inability to make meaningful comparisons they single out the sensationalist media for particular attention. The media, they argue, often conveys false images of relative risks through an emphasis on major events. There is, of course, an abundance of evidence to support the claim that media coverage of potentially hazardous situations or events is governed more by a need to excite the public than to inform or educate it. As Singer and Endreny discovered in their analysis of the way the media reports risk:

> what is newsworthy does not correspond very well with the distribution of hazards in the real world, as measured by mortality figures. Why not? Because, as it turns out, the media tend to feature…"catastrophic" accidents—accidents in which five or more people are killed simultaneously. Such accidents rank near or at the top of media attention, even though with one exception, automobile accidents, they do not result in a large number of deaths per year. Thus, media definitions of risk are based on the drama of the single hazardous event, not on the cumulatively greater but less spectacular risk reflected in annual mortality figures.[37]

Recognizing that bad news sells, the media tends to headline major accidents or natural disasters, even though these are low probability events. That is, single events in which large numbers of people are killed are rare. When they do occur, the media seldom report how many people involved in such activity were "at risk" and yet were unharmed. Take, for example, an airline accident. Without downplaying the tragedy of, say, 100 people dying in an airplane crash, the fact is that tens of thousands of passengers are safely transported through the sky daily. Thus, to calculate the chances of losing your life in a plane crash, you need to consider not only how many persons die from participation but also how many were at risk.

Urquhart and Heilmann developed a scale for measuring risks that is similar to the Richter scale for measuring the intensity of earthquakes. The units in their measure are given as *safety degree units* (SDU) because they wanted to emphasize the safety of certain hazards as well as the risks. For example, the risks of cigarette smoking is placed at 2.8 SDU while the risk of being struck by lightening is 7.0 SDU. Clearly, then, there is a much greater likelihood that you will end up in the morgue through smoking than being hit by a bolt of lightening.[38]

While the safety-degree scale may give us a practical way to measure and compare competing risks of death, one will not be able to make decisions based on it alone. Consider again the examples of being a passenger in an airplane or being a passenger in an automobile. Their respective safety-degree values are 3.6 and 5.9. Can an individual, simply on the basis of this information, determine whether he or she should fly or drive? Of course not. Many other factors enter into our decision-making process with respect to selecting a mode of transportation—monetary and temporal costs, convenience and comfort, desire to go sightseeing, to name but a few. In other words, once we *know* the calculated risks, we still have to decide (and this is where the other factors come into play) whether we are willing to *take* the risk. As we have noted, the ***perception of risk*** varies considerably from one individual (and situation) to another. Thus, in Urquhart and Heilman's calculus, lightening, which kills less than one person for every million exposed, has a safety degree of more than six. Motorcycling, on the other hand, which kills one in a thousand, rates only a three. In other words, it is much more dangerous to ride a motorcycle. Yet, the two risks are not perceived in that fashion. Death by a lightening strike is viewed as the greater risk by many. As risk analysts have repeatedly shown, perception often has little to do with reality.

Another problem with the indicator is that it does not help in areas where the death rate for a given hazard is not known. In a later chapter, for example, we will note that the Environmental Protection Agency seldom evaluates the synergy of two or more pesticides used together, so that the potential dangers of such chemical interactions are not known. Moreover, the scale could become another tool to be misused by industries attempting to cloud the facts about the danger of their product.

If used properly, the safety degree scale could benefit communities that are trying realistically to weigh the facts of different hazards so that they can choose the best alternative. Instead of leaving the decision up to distanced government officials, who may have political or other ulterior motives, each group at risk could be identified and given a clear and simple choice. The citizens of Tacoma, Washington faced such a decision in 1983 in relation to whether a copper smelting industry should stay or go. They had no precise comparative measures of the risks involved. In this case the head of the Environmental Protection Agency left the resolution of the issues to the community. There was considerable debate over the decision whether or not to close the smelting plant and, whether it was fair to give the community the right to struggle over such a controversial issue. In the end, the plant closed and the people of Tacoma were generally relieved of the burden of regulation. In a later chapter we shall examine in greater detail emerging citizen\community initiatives in dealing with such issues.

An important lesson was learned from the Tacoma incident. Given adequate information about a given risk, people seem willing to make tradeoffs and decide for themselves on matters of life and death. Again, it is presumed that with such information available people can make the personal decisions necessary for lengthening their own lives when faced with a hazardous environment. However, before this information can be easily conveyed there must be clear definitions of the risks involved and a way to measure them.

Health Risk Appraisal Programs. Illustrative of such attempts are a variety of health risk appraisal programs (HRAs). Hundreds of such programs have evolved as part of the growing interest in preventive medicine. They are used for health education purposes or to stimulate changes in health behavior. A review of over 200 programs notes that the rapid expansion of health risk appraisals is due to several factors:

> HRA is a relatively simple device that carries an implicit association with medical science; it is self-administered; it can use simple physiologic measures; it has utility for application to large groups as well as in one-on-one counseling; it is easily programmed to a variety of computer applications; and, it is relatively inexpensive.[39]

Several models for risk computation have been developed to assess the probabilities of major illnesses and diseases, such as coronary diseases, stroke, and traumatic injury.

HRA is a technique which compares an individual's health-related behavior and personal characteristics with mortality and epidemiological data as well as information on family history and personal behavior patterns. From this intricate analysis are derived estimates of the risk of dying at a particular age.

Estimates of the amount of risk that could be eliminated by appropriate behavioral changes are also computed. A key element is the provision of helpful feedback to the individual in the form of a personal *risk profile*.

Many have found HRAs a useful tool for setting priorities for getting healthier and living longer. They typically indicate your particular risk for certain diseases relative to average risk. You might learn, for example, that you have a 15 percent probability of having a heart attack, compared with an average risk of 5 percent for persons your age and sex. Lifestyle changes may be recommended in order to reduce the odds of an early trip to the grave. On the other hand, questions have been raised about the generalizability of these risk appraisals because of the problem of extrapolating from population data to statements about individuals. This is known to demographers and others as the *ecological fallacy*. The approach may not sufficiently take into account a person's unique genetic strengths and weaknesses. There are, apparently, "many people with devil-may-care health habits or ominous family histories (who) still live long, healthy lives."[40] Moreover, there again is the assumption that furnishing people with relevant information will lead them to modify their behavior in order to reduce the possibilities of illness and premature death. We have ample evidence that large numbers of people lack the motivation to change, or refuse to alter their lifestyle, even when confronted with information that their current living patterns are detrimental to their health. More than one investigator has noted that, "there is ample evidence that individuals confronted with risky choices do not behave in accordance with purely rational calculations of benefits and costs."[41]

The fact is that most of us are irrational when it comes to weighing the probabilities of risk. Being aware, for example, that we are thirteen times as likely to be hit by lightening as to win the lottery jackpot, does not prevent us from purchasing those promising tickets or repeatedly entering contests where the chances of winning often have odds of millions to one. The concept of *risk homeostasis*, further informs of the irrational side of the human character. The concept derives from the postulate "that people tend to embrace a certain level of risk. When something is made safer, they will somehow reassert the original level of danger."[42] It has been observed, for example, that after roads have been improved by more and wider lanes, people feel safer and subsequently drive faster. It does not occur to them that by doing so, that is, by reasserting the original risk level; they cancel out the benefits that improved roads confer.

Health-risk appraisal programs also raise a number of ethical questions. For example: Is *actively* seeking behavior modification an ethically acceptable stance for medical practitioners or employers?" Today hundreds of companies use health-risk appraisals to gauge the condition of their employees and to promote better health through programs that emphasize smoking cessation, weight reduction, nutrition information, exercise, and so on.[43] Is behavior modification an ethical goal for any group or agency concerned with people's well being and, if so, where do we draw the line between information and *coercion*?

That the potential for intimidation exists was illustrated in an editorial from the *New York Times* concerning cases of what has been termed *life-style discrim-*

ination.[44] In one case a woman was fired from her job when traces of nicotine were found in her urine. In a second case a man was dismissed from his company after admitting that he had consumed alcoholic beverages several years earlier. In both instances there was an absolute, inviolable company policy against smoking or drinking—ever. The clash between employee rights to privacy and company prerogatives to regulate lifestyles calls attention to a basic conflict. It is a conflict not easily resolved except perhaps through legal action.

The growing health consciousness of the general public increasingly brings into focus this contention between individual prerogatives and societal concerns. Cases involving so-called "pregnancy police", dramatically illustrate this confrontation of values.[45] In the past many women would smoke or drink throughout their pregnancies with little or no concern voiced by the public. However, that sort of "live and let live" attitude is changing. In a Gallup poll nearly half of the people questioned agreed that a woman who smoked or consumed alcoholic drinks during her pregnancy should be liable for damages to the baby. An expanding public consciousness of the connection between lifestyle habits and pregnancy outcomes, such as fetal alcoholic syndrome and crack babies "has prompted law-enforcement officials and ordinary citizens alike to intervene in what was once considered the most private realm of a woman's life"(p.52). In one such incident two cocktail waitresses informed a pregnant customer of their disapproval of her consuming alcohol and their reluctance to serve her. Even though some praised them for this action, they were fired for what others perceived to be rudeness.

People are beginning to challenge a person's right to privacy in matters of health. Since the mid-1980s criminal charges, such as child abuse, assault and manslaughter, have been brought against a growing number of pregnant drug addicts. While in the majority of instances the courts have supported the mother's right to privacy, the scales of justice are shifting in the face of mounting evidence of the deleterious effects of drugs and alcohol on fetal health and survival.

Attitudes and Risk-Taking

We have noted that many (maybe most?) people, when made aware that they are engaged in behavior that is detrimental to their health or is life-threatening, continue to resist altering their approach to living. Such defiance leads us to recognize that attitudes play a significant role in defining our vulnerability to life-threatening conditions or situations and how we react to them. Indeed, in many instances one's basic attitudes toward life determine the kinds of risks one is willing to take. Our newspapers and magazines are filled with reports of persons who **voluntarily** placed themselves in positions of heightened danger. A bizarre example is the man who attached 42 helium balloons to a lawn chair for an unorthodox flight over Long Beach, California.[46] In the same story that reported this unusual activity we are told a somewhat more familiar episode about a woman skydiver whose parachute failed to open, leading her to crash into the ground at more than 70 miles per hour. Upon being interviewed she indicates that she felt the risks of skydiving are worth it and that she will continue to jump. She wants to become the best woman skydiver in the world.

Less dramatic but equally dangerous are the so-called "free soloist" rock climbers who scale heights *without* the usual protections against falls. Instead they rely primarily on the strength of their handholds and finger tips to make the obviously dangerous ascent to the top. One such solo climber is quoted as saying: "Death is so close…You could let go and make the decision to die. It feels so good."[47] Rock climbing has enjoyed an unprecedented surge of popularity in recent years, and with it have come fatal accidents in which the climber slips and plunges hundreds of feet to the ground.

Why such people feel compelled to risk their lives and "test the will to live" is not readily apparent. Some suggest that such people take risks because they are frustrated over things that affect them and over which they feel they have no control, such as changes in the economy, or government rules and regulations that impinge on their personal lives. Hence, they engage in dangerous activity in order to emphasize or reassert their individuality, rather than simply being treated as just another number. In this view: "Risk-taking is something over which they have control. If they conquer a mountain or jump out of a plane, they've proved something. They've gotten the thrill of a conquest, and proved they are unusual, different from other people."[48] Individuals who "spiderman" their way up some of our tallest city buildings, or parachute off the top of them, would certainly fall into this category. So would those people, featured in a television program titled **The Extreme Edge**. Among others, the program highlighted a man who took one, deep breath, and then dove between 328 and 344 feet below the water, subjecting his body to more than a hundred tons of pressure. Also portrayed were individuals engaged in dry land *luge*, which involves lying on one's back on a roller board, feet forward, pushing off and eventually achieving speeds of 70 miles per hour or more, racing downhill over eight miles, with fifty turns, of paved southern California roads. The only "brakes" available are treaded sneakers or shoes that one drags along the ground. Even in the Olympic competitions, with all their precautions, luging is generally considered a "daredevil" sport.

A more common explanation of why people take such risks, or push the limits of potentially dangerous activity, is that certain behaviors simply are ways of expressing our adventurous spirit. Some people engage in such activity primarily for the thrill of it. This may especially be the case with respect to certain recreational activities and sports; for example, jumping out of airplanes to skydive, whitewater kayaking, race car driving, scuba diving, motorcycle racing, para-sailing, cave-diving, and mountain climbing. The attraction of bungee jumping, in which people leap from buildings, bridges, and other heights while tethered to reinforced elastic ropes, no doubt derives from the anticipated thrill and exhilaration of falling through space. The potential for damage to the body or for accidents apparently is not sufficient discouragement for many people.

Even in the case of many recreational sports, the risks and dangers to limb and life are often underestimated. Take, example, those who ski down mountainsides. This exhilarating type of recreation carries with it the potential for great injury. At Vail, the well-known resort in Colorado, a least a hundred skiers a day are treated at the hospital emergency center during the peaks of the season. Multiply this by similar occurrences at other resorts across the nation and you get some idea of the widespread prevalence of such incidents. In fact, skiing casualty counts are increasing across the country. Along with that upswing has come a noticeable rise in serious and catastrophic injuries, and fatalities. Most casual skiers are relatively uninformed as to how to protect themselves from potential danger, thereby failing to minimize the risk of injury or death in gliding down the mountain They usually do not know, for example which skis are the best and safest for their level of skiing, or understand how or why bindings work. Nor do they typically know how to fall, or what the proper settings are for release. Moreover, many do not have adequate understanding of skiing protocols and what dangers can ensue when they are violated. The skiing industry has been criticized for being more concerned with its image and profits than emphasizing safety factors and techniques, for concealing the true risks involved, and for treating the injury factor as an irrelevancy. One critic argues that the prevailing attitude is "that the sport is "naturally dangerous," and therefore to participate you must learn to live with it, and please remove the bodies before they despoil the view."[49] Many people learn, too late, that skiing can be a risky venture.

That the majority of these venturesome types are young should come as no surprise. The young are especially apt to place themselves in life-threatening situations. Lacking the social and psychological maturity that eventually comes with age and experience, they often exhibit a bravado accompanied by a feeling of invulnerability in the face of danger. They are susceptible to challenges and dares which, if accepted, carry with them the real possibility of serious accidents—even death. As I write this, our local paper reports the demise of a 21 year old university student who went out for an evening of hard drinking with his roommates. He had accepted their challenge to break their record for downing shots of alcohol. Within one hour he had put away 23 drinks of various types, then became violently ill, and subsequently passed out. Taken to the hospital, he died early the next morning of complications of *acute **ethanol intoxication**.*[50] The head of the student's major department on campus noted the sad irony that this event took place only a few hours after a national network television program dealing with the problem of young drinkers. It highlighted the case of a 15 year old that drank himself to death on a vodka binge.

The program also included a segment on alcoholic abuse on college campuses. Abusive drinking is defined by the National Institute of Drug Abuse as the consumption of five or more drinks at one sitting. College administrators generally agree that while the pattern of abusive drinking among college students has remained fairly stable over the past decade, ***binge* drinking** is increasing. More cases like the following are being reported in the nation's newspapers:

Isaac and Alease Parsons had warned their son Wayne, a 19-year-old sophomore at Virginia Tech, about the perils of alcohol…he had even been lectured to by an older brother. But when Wayne went to a party with about 30 other people at a friend's apartment one night…he gulped a large quantity of beer, then in 15 minutes drank an oversized tumbler of about 32 ounces of tequila…About an hour later, he collapsed. An emergency medical crew was called but could not revive him. He died in the hospital…the next morning.[51]

Like the previous case, it was again determined that the cause of death was alcohol poisoning. College students are not totally unaware of the life-threatening potential of binge drinking, especially where such incidents have occurred on their own campuses. Given that awareness, why do they engage in such death-defying behavior anyway? Is it a reflection of youthful innocence or a sense of invulnerability? Does this activity indicate overconfidence that one can judge when the dangerous limit is being approached and have enough control to stop? Excessive drinking among today's college students has been attributed to rising peer and academic pressures. Some contend that they also are confronted with many more difficulties than previous generations, including easy exposure to alcohol, risky sexual behavior, and an uncertain economy. Among the myriad of possible explanations, the influence of peer pressure gets repeatedly mentioned.

Peer pressure can be viewed as part of normal development in the maturation process.[52] However, it can also be a major source of the development of risk-taking behavior, including violence and substance abuse.[53] As one can see, the consequences of acquiescing to those pressures, or accepting their challenges, can have lethal consequences.

There are, of course, many other reasons why certain individuals take unnecessary risks. Some, for example, may be reflecting what has been depicted as a thrill-seeking personality type. Others may choose to engage in such activities because of the personal challenge they pose to their confidence and ability to overcome physical and emotional obstacles. A. Alvarez, author and psychiatrist, was quoted in the *New York Times Magazine* as saying:

> the pleasure of risk is in the control needed to ride it with assurance so that what appears dangerous to the outside is, to the participant, simply a matter of intelligence, skill, intuition, coordination—in a word, experience. Climbing, in particular, is a paradoxically intellectual pastime, but with this difference: you have to think with your body. Every move has to be worked out in terms of effort, balance and consequences. It is like playing chess with your body. If I make a mistake, the consequences are immediate, obvious, embarrassing and possibly painful. For a brief period, I am directly responsible for my actions. In that beautiful, silent world of the mountains, it seems to me worth a little risk.

Still others derive excitement and satisfaction *because* there is an element of danger, and from successfully achieving the goal involved. There seems to be general agreement that many risk takers are **stimulus addictive**—they experience a special form of ecstasy from living on the brink of danger. They often speak of getting a unique "high" from voluntary exposure to potentially dangerous conditions. They can clearly recall such situations, in which they experienced vivid moments of exhilaration from the potent mixture of excitement and fear.

The majority of participants in risk-taking recreation readily acknowledge the potential dangers inherent in these activities, and take the necessary precautions. But others are not so cautious, and take on additional risks that place their lives in jeopardy. DeSpelder and Strickland[54] give the following illustration:

> Although mountain climbing involves obvious risks, two different climbers may relate to them in vastly different ways. One may begin the climb with an attitude of abandon that could only be characterized as foolhardy or death defying. The other may devote many hours to obtaining instructions, preparing equipment, conditioning for the climb, and asking advice from more

experienced climbers before setting foot on the mountain. In short, steps can be taken to minimize the risks. An activity, then, may be attractive to some persons *because* of its inherent risks, whereas others accept the risks as inseparable from the other attractive features of the activity.

Thus, in the case of the first climber, the individual ignores common sense and fails to make the necessary preparations whereby, if the situation demanded, he could exercise options that would allow him to manage or control the element of risk. In the case of the second climber, precautions have been taken to minimize the potential hazards. Unfortunately, many otherwise intelligent people assume that little experience is necessary for participating in such endeavors. Each year, for example, well over a thousand people register to climb Mt. McKinley in Alaska. Its fierce stormy weather, extremely thin altitude, and difficult accessibility make it one of the world's most dangerous mountains. Over the years at least 80 people have perished in attempts to climb to its peak. Many attempt to do so with little or no experience, without a guide, or lacking proper equipment. A Park Service volunteer who operates the base camp radio commented that: "It seems like the ones with the least experience are the ones with the most summit fever."[55] She goes on to describe one foolhardy individual who arrived at the base camp without crampons or a parka, toting all his gear in a shopping bag. He ignored her pleas to not proceed, and started up the glacier alone. Fortunately, a Park Service Ranger eventually turned him back—but only after he had somehow succeeded in climbing to the 14,000 foot level! Such people often evidence a "do or die" attitude, and their persistence in the face of danger has necessitated frequent high altitude rescues. Attitudes do make a difference. As William James once noted: "The greatest discovery of my generation is that a human being can alter his life by altering his attitude." Many have died prematurely for failing to follow that sage advice.

Faith and Fatalism. Our attitudes regarding our mortality, indeed, our philosophy of life in general, influence how we attend to our health and survival. Some individuals treat danger with greater equanimity than others. For example, a person with a strong faith in the promises of a better life in the hereafter is apt to be less afraid of mortal peril than one who perceives death as the final extinction. An attitude of *fatalism*, which conditions people to accept passively whatever may befall them, can lower their guard against danger. Their basic attitude is "what will be will be." Such a stance tends to place them in a particularly risky position. It keeps their guard down and makes their existence unnecessarily vulnerable to the dangers and life-threatening elements in their environment. If one believes that we are mere pawns of fate, one is apt to be more susceptible to threats of injury or death.[56]

Often, such people attribute the outcome of life events to *luck*. Trusting in luck, however, often leads them to take chances with their health by clinging to harmful habits, such as excessive drinking or smoking. Underlying this nonchalance is the fatalistic belief that when "your number is up," there is nothing that you can do about it. Television inundates us with the effects of war and violence and for many young people; in particular, daily events lead them to adapt the deadly slogan of Pretty Boy Romano, the troubled youngster in the old Humphrey Bogart movie <u>Knock on Any Door</u>: "Live fast, die young, and have a good looking corpse." This sort of cavalier attitude is reinforced by the human sense of uniqueness: "If anybody can beat the odds, I can." Of course, few gamblers ever remain in the win column.

No one, of course, would deny that luck sometimes plays a role in the course of our lives. We all know people who have avoided injury or premature death through one or more unplanned but fortunate set of chance circumstances or events. Upon closer scrutiny, however, what appears to outsiders as luck more often than not turns out to be simply the result of *good planning*. "Hope for nothing from luck," Edward Bulwer-Lytton wrote, "and the probability is that you will be so prepared, forewarned, and forearmed that all shallow observers will call you lucky."[57] So-called lucky people, it turns out, move through life with a set of attitudes that enhance the probabilities of success—by preparing for their "breaks," and by developing habits that capitalize on good fortune. Above all, they do not depend on its fortuitous appearance in order to achieve successful living, or to avoid disasters, or, to put this in more colloquial terms, to save their skins in moments of crisis. "Lucky people know the difference between risky and rash, between an informed hunch and vain hope."[58] In short, leaving things to chance is not ordinarily part of their daily repertoire.

They do, however, take risks. They recognize, like most of us do, that the excelsior of life would probably disappear if all chance-taking were totally removed from daily living. For example, we ordinarily would not forego a vacation abroad because of the possibility that the plane might crash. Nor would an avid sportsman decline an invitation to accompany friends on a deep sea fishing venture for fear of the boat sinking. The fact is that no person can expect to a life totally devoid of taking chances. Who would want to, anyway? "To live at all is to live a little dangerously; to live in the fullest sense of the word is to balance personal fulfillment against risk."[59] In order to enhance our potential for survival, however, we need to avoid creating additional and unnecessary danger to our daily endeavors. One must routinely ask whether the added hazard is worth it. For example, given the known risks of exceeding the speed limit, is the benefit of arriving at one's destination sooner worth the danger of having an accident?

The fact is that many widely accepted human activities are fraught with the potential for damaging our bodies or even killing us.

> Spend an afternoon in an orthopedic clinic at the foot of a ski resort if you want to understand something about the risk of skiing. Spend a Saturday night in your local emergency room if you want to understand something about the risks of drinking and driving, drinking and fighting, and drinking and being a pedestrian. Spend a day in your local VD clinic if you want to understand something about the risks of sex with strangers—and sometimes with friends. These adverse outcomes have their origins in self-initiated activities, and they illustrate the principle that people will engage in fairly hair-raising activities on their own initiative, while steadfastly maintaining their right to protest vehemently when forced into something quite tame by comparison.[60]

The reasonably prudent person always seeks to distinguish between the risks that are realistic and those that are reckless or just plain silly. General George S. Patton Jr., who had an international reputation for being an outrageous risk-taker, once wrote: "Take calculated risks. That is quite different from being rash." And, one might similarly add, that is quite different from swashbuckling recklessness or pathogenic fearlessness.

Calculated risks imply, in part, a conscious attempt to minimize the degree of uncertainty in confronting the unknown or dangerous situations. A good example here is Charles Lindbergh's historic and incredible solo flight across the Atlantic Ocean in a small, single engine plane. That daring and heroic act earned him, among other things, the nickname "Lucky Lindy." However, his accomplishment had little to do with happenstance. He was a thoroughly experienced pilot and mechanic who carefully assessed the practicalities of his plane being able to traverse safely that long a distance. Months of concentrated effort, during which he oversaw every detail of his plane's construction and calculated every aspect of the trip, preceded the actual day of departure. It is largely for these reasons that he was able to land in Paris not only ahead of schedule but did so with sufficient fuel to continue another 1000 miles. Similarly, our modern astronauts leave little to chance on their flights into the stratosphere and to the moon. Those adventures into space involve incredible numbers of hours of preparation before, during, and after each mission—all calculated to minimize errors and the probabilities of things going wrong. Even then, as the tragic events surrounding the explosion of the Challenger rocket painfully remind us, an overlooked problem (remember the "O" rings?) and errors of judgment on the part of others involved in the final decision to launch, can lead to devastation and the loss of lives.

One can perhaps never completely eliminate uncertainty, nor would one necessarily want to. Indeed, it has been observed that: "It was the search for the good things in life while risking the bad that set people on the road to civilization. If they had wanted a maximum of certainty in their lives, they might never have emerged from the caves."[61] Few would disagree with the argument that only through a constant willingness to confront the unknown is humankind able to move forward. Similarly, at the individual level, there is considerable consensus that high achievers are often people who are willing to engage in risky pursuits that might result in failure. Some well-known personalities fit into this category, for example: H. Ross Perot, a self-made billionaire, who in the 1980s organized a daring raid to free some employees from a Tehran prison; Dick Rutan and Jeana Yeager, who successfully completed a bruising nine-day, nonstop flight around the world in a feather-light aircraft without refueling. One can think of many others. While the motivations for becoming involved in life-endangering situations may vary, a common approach appears to be evident among these and other high achievers. They make careful plans, consider all the relevant contingencies, and take the necessary precautions. When confronted with a decision to act in the face of uncertainty they strive to achieve a balance between the competing inclinations of boldness and prudence. This is a delicate balance, but one that is essential in eliminating preventable risks while guiding the "questing spirit" of human beings.[62]

2

Personality Attributes and Survival

The Role of Attitudes and Values

We have noted that there is a wide range of contexts in which attitudes serve to increase or decrease human vulnerability. They are often subtle and difficult to identify, but nevertheless powerful components of our life-and-death styles.

Machismo. Attitudes frequently are closely related to the culture or subculture in which we are embedded. Illustrative here are those pertaining to gender role definitions and expectations, and in particular those that involve traditional notions, for example, of *machismo* in the face of traumatic events. Society expects males to "be real men," to fend for themselves, to be self-reliant and to avoid becoming dependent, and to conquer successfully personal and impersonal challenges without emotional involvement. However, they are not always able to live up to this expectation. Yet the felt pressure to follow a "stiff upper lip" philosophy in the face of adversity may lead to isolation, a diminished capacity to cope, and a heightened vulnerability.[63] In this sense males become victims of what is sometimes referred to as the masculine mystique or the masculine must be strong ethic.

The expectation that men play a stoic, nonemotional role even in the face of crises can have negative consequences. Adherence to this definition of masculinity may prove deleterious to the emotional and physical health of the man as he encounters stress. Such stress is often apparent during the so-called midlife crisis, where he faces a series of adjustments related to the beginnings of bodily decline, career stagnation, and changes within his family unit. Safely traversing late life transitions, such as a change in marital status due to the loss of a spouse, can become particularly problematic if one attempts to strictly adhere to a masculine ethic characteristic of earlier generations. In my own study of older widowers, for example, it was noted that:

18

...society expects males to fend for themselves and avoid being dependent. This is an expectation that the widower is not always quite able to live up to. But his *awareness* of that expectation may lead to a certain hesitation or reluctance to ask for or seek assistance. Indeed, this awareness may sometimes make the widower feel compelled to sustain an image of self-sufficiency in the face of a burdensome existence...for some widowers, isolation and loneliness are the consequences of this reluctance to admit an inability to maintain a rewarding independent existence.[64]

The result often is an increased vulnerability to the vicissitudes of later life and a growing inability to fend off the stress of involuntary social isolation.

The "strong, silent type," who often tensely persists in projecting the image of a nondisclosing persona, may also pay a heavy price for his machismo in the form of a shorter life span. "Macho men eventually suffer failed relationships and aborted careers. They may also wind up physically crippled or dead at an early age from hypertension, coronary artery disease or a variety of other illnesses." Some psychologists have observed that this type of male frequently ignores his personal health, tends to take more risks than usual in driving or sports, represses emotional expression, and often reacts to stress by overeating, drinking or smoking. By denying his vulnerability, he is pretending he is immortal. His body, of course, has no such illusions.

Such negative outcomes are not, of course, inevitable. They can be avoided by de-emphasizing strict adherence to the machismo elements of masculinity. This means abandoning harmful attitudes of that male ethic, such a fear of dependency, in favor of other dimensions such as interdependency. It also includes a willingness to be open to change, to admit to one's be more emotional responsiveness, to place greater emphasis and value on interpersonal relations and networking. At the same time, one can retain some of the positive attitudes of the male ethic, characterized by a heavy emphasis on being forthright, non-manipulative, and a concern with integrity.

Cynicism. Early evidence exists of other personality attributes which apparently have the potential to hasten our demise. In the 1950s two cardiologists, Meyer Friedman and Ray Rosenman, discovered *Type A* personalities—a complex of behavioral dispositions exemplified by people who were hard-driving and competitive, aggressive, hostile, hurried, impatient, prone to interrupt others, who walked, talked, and ate quickly, and who drove themselves relentlessly as ambitious workaholics—were more likely to experience heart problems and heart attacks than their more subdued *Type B* counterparts. The type B personalities react to their environment without often feeling impatient or angry or with a chronic sense of urgency. They tend to be more relaxed and easy-going, readily satisfied and less concerned with achievement, a need to acquire more things, or always having to do everything in a hurry. Subsequent investigations in the United States and other countries supported these early findings and the attributes of the two types quickly drifted into popular usage.

However, several later studies failed to link conclusively Type A behavior with heart disease. Researchers suspected that one reason for this lack of supportive evidence might be that Type A was initially too broadly defined, and that certain of its negative components, such as those that measured hostility or anger, may be more predictive of heart problems than others. Consequently they administered a section of the widely used Minnesota Multiphasic Personality Inventory that measures these attributes to patients undergoing examinations for atherosclerotic symptoms. They found that patients with high levels of hostility were 50 percent more likely to have clogged arteries than patients who scored low.

In a related retrospective study, it was found that among physicians tested 25 years earlier, those with high hostility scores had *five times* more heart disease than others who scored below the median. Further analysis of the hostility measure revealed that it was mostly tapping an attitude of mistrust, that is, cynicism.[65] Moreover, experiments have shown that mistrustful people produce more 'fight-or-flight' hormones in various situations than do more trustful persons. Since these hormones are believed to accelerate plaque buildup on artery walls—"hardening" of the arteries—those who expected the worst from the world around them might find themselves leaving it sooner."[66] Indeed, recent studies indicate that the increased risk of heart disease associated with chronic hostility and cynicism is similar to that created by having high cholesterol or high blood pressure.

The experts in this area caution that being a workaholic, always being in a hurry, talking fast, interrupting, and so on, is not *necessarily* harmful to your heart. However, it is unhealthy if, in addition to these traits, you also have high levels of hostility and anger which you have difficulty bringing under control. It has been found, for example, that when persons with high hostility scores are subjected to experimental conditions that arouse mistrust of others and also provoke anger, they exhibit stronger blood pressure responses than people with low hostility scores. The consequences can be fatal. In one of the series of studies the scientists looked at the scores of a sample of lawyers who had taken a psychological test 25 years earlier. They found that during the interim the attorneys who had scored high on hostility on that test died at a rate more than four times that of peers with lower scores.

It is, of course, very difficult to eliminate persistent feelings of hostility and an attitude of distrust that has over time become a basic component of one's personality. Some people may be able to reduce the dangers of chronic cynicism through a program of behavior modification. Others may have to resort to drugs to block the offending hormones. In any event, if the goal is to strengthen one's survival potential, some modification of the cynical outlook appears essential. While changes in basic temperament are by no means easy to accomplish, it is possible to alter attitudes and feelings of mistrust, to diminish the frequency and intensity of angry outbursts, and to learn to treat others with greater consideration. Taking such steps may help avoid unnecessary illness and premature death.

Optimism. The mounting evidence that attitudinal modifications can have positive survival consequences led to a branch of medicine called ***psychoneuroimmunology***. It seeks to understand the physiological effects of attitudes and emotions by looking at the interactions between the brain, the endocrine system, and the immune system. Findings from psychoneuroimmunologic analyses suggest that strong positive attitudes can sometimes make a significant difference in a patient's ability to overcome illness—even life-threatening illness. It appears, for example, that affirmative emotions "actually can stimulate the spleen, producing an increase in red blood cells and a corresponding increase in the number of cancer-fighting cells. These cells can destroy the cancer cells one by one, leaving normal tissue untouched—unlike chemotherapy, which cannot distinguish between normal and malignant cells."[67] Evidence is mounting that particular emotions can affect our bodies and make a significant difference in our ability to overcome illness and, therefore, in the quality of our lives.

It is common for patients suffering from catastrophic illnesses to experience panic and helplessness that can lead to severe depression. Severe depression in turn tends to weaken the body's immune system. Research is beginning to show strategies of treatment designed to relieve that depression which, when successful, tend to enhance the immune system. This has led some to contend that: "All the positive forces—love, hope, faith, will to live, determination, purpose, festivity, laughter—are powerful antagonists of depression and help to create an environment that makes medical care more effective."[68] Let us look a little more closely at one of these common human emotions—laughter.

Laughter and Good Health. A good sense of humor may help keep us well and even recover from illness. Illustrative here is an experiment involving medical students who were tested for the amount of salivary immunoglobulin-A in their systems before and after seeing an amusing film. Immunoglobulin, an antibody used to defend against respiratory viral infections, showed a measurable increase following laughter. Laughter apparently boosts our immune system by decreasing the level of **cortisol**, an immune suppressor, in the body. It may also lower levels of **catecholamines**, hormones associated with stress. Again, experiments in which subjects watch a humorous videotape found they had lower blood levels of stress hormones, such as **epinephrine** and **dopamine**, than a control group that had not viewed the film.[69] Related studies have found that student apprehension over grades as examination dates drew close could impair their immune system, as reflected in a pronounced increase in colds and other illnesses. It appears that laughter also stimulates the *pituitary gland*, triggering the release of **endorphins** and **enkephalins**. These are natural painkillers that may relieve arthritis and other inflammatory pain.

It is important to point out that the hormonal changes being discussed here are all of a temporary nature. Subsequent to the experiments subjects' hormonal levels returned to normal. Humor alone, of course, cannot be a cure-all or work miracles. Nor is it a replacement for competent medical treatment. However, there is the suggestion here that people who regularly use humor as part of their repertoire for coping with everyday life may get longer-lasting benefits.

> Most experts believe that mirthful laughter, not sarcastic, put-down humor, is responsible for any benefits. Negative humor pushes people away from one another. Mirth stems from an enduring sense of humor. It builds warm, caring bonds between people, helps put problems in perspective and fosters a sense of joy in being alive.[70]

It appears that people who approach daily living with an attitude of playfulness, and who have cultivated a sense of delight in the human condition, who enjoy an uninhibited belly laugh, may in the process be promoting their own good health. One of the better known proponents of this mind-body connection was the late Norman Cousins, author and long-time editor of *The Saturday Evening Review*. As a result of his experiences in recovering from a serious illness he developed a strong interest in the newly named science of psychneuroimmunology.[71] He eventually joined the staff at the University of California School of Medicine as an adjunct professor in the department of psychiatry and biobehavioral sciences. The projects conducted there on the role of emotions in illness further convinced him that what you believe and feel can make a difference in your health. In various interviews he provided several examples of this connection. One interesting incident, which may ring familiar to some readers, affected hundreds of fans at a football game in Los Angeles.[72]

A half-dozen spectators became ill with food poisoning. The examining physician ascertained that all had consumed soft drinks from the dispensing machine under the stands. He directed that an announcement be made alerting people to the health hazards of the soft drinks, calling attention to the fact that some spectators had come down with food poisoning. Immediately, the stadium became a sea of retching and fainting people. Two hundred persons had to be hospitalized. Then it was ascertained that the soft drinks had nothing to do with the illness. When this fact became known, everyone's symptoms cleared up.

The entire episode, of course, was due to ***conversion hysteria***, a well documented process whereby psychosocial factors are transformed into actual illness. The imagination and emotions obviously play a real role here. To put this in slightly altered phraseology of an old sociological dictum: if you can imagine something as real, it may then become real in its consequences.

The operation of that dictum, especially in suggesting linkages between mind and body, is apparent in research which utilizes placebos (from the Latin, "I will please"). These are chemically inert or inactive substances, such as a sugar pill, that look like real medication but in fact are not. A typical experiment involves giving one group of subjects medication and a comparable group a placebo. However, both think they are getting the actual medication. The results indicate that the placebo often is as effective as the medication, suggesting the influence of subjective or psychological factors in the outcome. A dramatic demonstration of these influences was provided by a controversial experiment conducted in the late 1950s.[73] In that experiment, one group of patients underwent coronary-by-pass surgery. Another group of patients were also put under anesthetic, and an incision was made, but no actual operation was performed on the heart arteries. It was found that the coronary-by-pass was no more effective than the sham treatment. Some have suggested that current coronary by-pass surgery may similarly derive at least part of its success from the placebo effect. It has been observed that many by-pass patients experience considerable relief following their operation, even though their surgery did *not* improve ventricular function. Hence: "The operation's symbolic and metaphorical effects may thus account for much of the patients' relief from angina pain."[74]

The Mind\Body Controversy

Since the nineteen fifties the field of psychosomatic medicine, or the notion that some diseases originate in emotional distress, has increased its efforts to prove this connection.[75] Today the idea that the mental images we produce may subtly change our emotions, in turn creating either a positive or a negative effect on our immune systems is widely accepted. Consequently, therapists are encouraging their clients to engage in positive "coping imagery" exercises during periods of stress in order to bolster their immunity.[76] Implicit here is a major assumption, namely, that it is possible for people to *summon* positive attitudes or emotions as an act of will to create a desired physiological effect. It is, in fact, a controversial assumption, and one that many are not willing to support until a broader scientific base is established which more strongly and directly corroborates these mind-body connections.

Findings from some studies in fact, challenge the assumption that a positive mental attitude can help prevent or cure a variety of illnesses. For example, researchers at the University of Pennsylvania Cancer Center gathered data from patients with advance cancer and others who had been treated either for breast cancer or melanoma and were susceptible to a recurrence of the disease.[77] These patients were asked about such attitudes as satisfaction with their jobs and life in general, feelings about their health, and their degree of helplessness and hopelessness—factors which some studies have shown to affect longevity. Three and a half years after this study began, 75 percent of the advanced cancer patients had died, and 26 percent of the people treated for melanoma or breast cancer had recurrences. However, no relationship between the positive or negative attitudes, and either the survival or recurrence rate could be found. In general, the more cheerful subjects showed no greater capacity than the depressed ones for fighting their cancers, and the pessimists were not at greater risk of death or recurrence than the optimists. In the words of the investigators, this study "suggests that the inherent biology of the disease alone determines the prognosis, overriding the potentially mitigating influences of psychosocial factors." As so often happens, this study was attacked for certain methodological shortcomings and for ignoring other evidence which supports the effectiveness of positive thinking in fighting disease, even life-threatening disease such as cancer.

Part of the problem is that the impact of the connection between mental states and emotional factors in illness is not a direct cause-and-effect relationship. It has been observed, for example, that despite the success of health practitioners in utilizing imaging techniques to overcome disease and to treat a wide variety of disorders, (depressions, insomnia, sexual dysfunction, asthma, and fibroid tumors) little is actually known about *why* or *how* mental imaging affects the immune system. Nevertheless, the strong suspicion remains that emotions may form the primary link between mind and immunity. A well known surgeon,[78] for example, posits that cancer is despair experienced at the cellular level. "If we ignore our despair," he writes, "the body receives a die message, If we deal with our pain and seek help, then the message is 'Living is difficult but desirable' and the immune system works to keep us alive."

This belief that a positive mental attitude is required for a successful battle against cancer (and other life-threatening diseases) has been criticized for the burden of guilt it places on the patient for failing to use personal will power to achieve a cure. Some assert that the message of many medical self-help books, is "if treatment fails, you have nobody to blame but yourself."[79] Sontag also takes issues with the premise of popular immunology, noting: "The hypothesis that distress can affect immunological responsiveness and in some circumstances lower immunity to disease is hardly the same as, or constitutes evidence for—the view that emotions *cause* disease, much less for the belief that specific emotions can produce specific diseases."[80] She and others are generally opposed to the currently popular holistic and alternative therapies, which are based in part upon the premises of psychoneuroimmunology, and which seek to enlist the patient's will to resist disease.

While this scientific controversy continues, the public appears to be increasingly receptive to the concept that interactions between the brain and the immune system can affect our health and our longevity. The long held belief that states of mind influence the susceptibilities of the body is gaining contemporary legitimacy as modern research techniques unravel these complex relationships.[81] Mental-imagery techniques, biofeedback programs, and the like have gained in popularity. The belief that mind-body connections are real, and real in their consequences, has apparently taken hold in the American consciousness.

The Will to Live. That we can exert *some* influence over the timing of our death through the exercise of will power has been demonstrated by analyses which reveal a so-called *death dip* before certain ceremonial occasions, often followed by a *death peak*.[82] That is to say, there is evidence that fewer deaths than expected occur prior to certain domestic, political, or religious events—such as birthdays, presidential elections, and the Jewish Day of Atonement. The death rates of Chinese-Americans are consistently lower before the annual Harvest Moon Festival and higher afterwards. Some additional evidence of a death-dip before the Olympic Games at the sites where they are held, and before Thanksgiving, have also been reported. Still others have documented a decline in suicide and total mortality levels during the months preceding presidential elections.[83]

These findings suggest some support for the folk wisdom that certain people near death can cling to life to reach an important event. Such instances seem to indicate that the mind is able to overcome the body—if only temporarily.[84] In a subsequent chapter we will note the other side of this coin, namely, the will to die. That is, people apparently can decide that they no longer wish to continue living under their present circumstances and, without obvious evidence of physical illness, proceed to expire, again giving some credence to the mind-body connection. In a later chapter dealing with the effects of stress on our health and life chances we shall again take up the implications of the field of psychoneuroimmunology.

Risk-Taking Personalities

The question as to why some people actively pursue risky endeavors that may result in failure, injury or even death, while others adhere to more conventional existences is difficult to answer. While there are several theories on why some individuals prefer to live dangerously, the reasons are often rooted in basic personality traits.

Some risk takers have been characterized as evidencing Type T (thrill seeking) personalities. Frank Farley, who originated the term, contends such people are driven by temperament to a life of constant stimulation, change and risk taking. They characteristically reject rules and regulations while pursuing the unknown or the uncertain. He estimates that these creative risk takers comprise as much as 30 percent of the general population. On the other hand, his own research revealed that Type T's had twice as many automobile accidents as non-Ts, and that many purposely drove while intoxicated for the additional excitement and risk.[85] Farley suspects that these personality types have a physical or genetic predisposition toward risk taking. In his view these people need and thrive on the uncertainty involved in stretching boundaries or taking chances, whether it be in the financial marketplace or flying highly experimental aircraft.[86]

A large array of social and sociopsychological factors may play a role in the development of risk taking personalities, including family environments and relationships. It appears that growing up in either a distressed family situation, one that has experienced various difficulties, *or* one that is highly nutrient and supportive, and at the same time maintains a pattern of high expectations for its members, *both* have the potential for producing people who are willing to engage in daring ventures. They possess a number of traits, such as—intelligence; intense persistence—even in the face of prior failure; a high degree of self-confidence; the capability to handle stress; often a strong religious faith—which may give them a sense of security and self-esteem; an attitude that control can be exercised to minimize failure by taking precautions ("The ones who succeed are those who don't jump off the bridge until they know the parachute works"); decisiveness; a strong drive for autonomy; adventuresome; ambitious; an inner restlessness; competitiveness; a high need for achievement and, in some instances, a desire to surpass the accomplishments of one's father.

The above list, of course, is far from comprehensive,[87] and says little about a host of cultural influences which promote and reward risk taking, such as money, honor, and prestige. "A democratic form of government emphasizing accomplishments of the individual further encourages a culture that can tolerate, and even encourage, risk takers."[88] One can make a case that American society values those individuals willing to "go for it," to risk "the whole ball of wax" in the pursuit of certain acceptable goals. While there may be some consensus that factors such as those mentioned above often characterize personalities with risk taking tendencies, we lack adequate instruments for measuring the exact degree to which each contributes—singly or in combination—to a pattern of taking chances.

Personality and Lethal Behavior

Many of the types of personalities discussed in the preceding section are apt to take what we referred to earlier as calculated risks, where an effort has been made to minimize failure or danger. Other types of personalities, however, exhibit a greater likelihood of placing themselves in hazardous circumstances. Numerous efforts have been made to identify the personality attributes associated with the propensity to take perilous risks. Using a psychosocial perspective, one team of investigators developed a lethal behavior scale and administered it to people of varying ages.[89] Not surprisingly, they found that young males were most likely to engage in such behaviors. They attribute this finding to certain personality traits which are most commonly, but not exclusively found in this category of people. The four traits found to correlate most strongly with lethal behavior were; a) an orientation toward danger—preference for violence in television and movies, participation in dangerous sports, etc., b) an orientation towards bravery and adventure, c) thrill seeking—fast driving and more accidents, and d) unsafe habits—not wearing seat belts, driving unsafely, and smoking. Interestingly, no significant difference in lethal behaviors were found between educational groups.

The lethal behaviors scale provides some insight into which categories of people might benefit most from education about risk-taking behaviors. A more specific indicator is needed to identify, not groups, but individuals who are most likely to fall into the risk category. In an effort to develop such a tool Keinan and

Meir[90] constructed a scale derived from an inventory to assess personality characteristics. The perspective underlying this scale holds that risky actions are part of
a lifestyle rather than spontaneous actions arising out of situational variables.
They were able to identify the following traits: 1) sensation seeking—the need for
stimulation through danger; 2) a high activity level; 3) low self control—often
acting on impulse; 4) a high degree of activity; (5) independence—struggles
against norms that impinge personal freedoms; and 6) a short-term time perspective. Tests of this scale on a variety of respondents indicate it is a reliable and valid
instrument for identifying persons who tend to seek adventure, tension, and risk.
There are a variety of uses for this information. For example, the results can be
employed to select participants in high risk jobs or assignments in the armed services. Another use is, of course, education. If people with a tendency toward
excessive risk-taking can be identified, then they can be made aware of their traits
and assisted in changing their lifestyle, if they so desire.

Personality traits probably affect the way an individual perceives the alternatives of a given situation. However, the decision as to whether or not to take a
risk involves more than these traits. There are, for example, various motives
which influence the way a person selects a particular pattern of action from a possible set of alternatives. Motives are dispositions "to strive for a certain kind of
satisfaction" and may be oriented towards maximizing satisfaction or minimizing
pain.[91] In addition to motives, the role of genetic predispositions must also be
taken into account.

The Biological Basis of Risk-Taking

Many scientists believe that there is a strong biological urge that propels risk takers to seek higher levels of stimulation in everything ranging from stock-market
speculation or sky diving to alcohol abuse or the tendency toward physical violence. Certain anthropologists, for example, argue that the propensity to take
risks can be traced to our hunting-gathering past and is deeply rooted in our biological make-up. Many believe a significant proportion of such behavior can be
traced to important genetic components. Thus, anthropologist Melvin Konner
stressed the influence of heredity, in noting that (a) a substantial proportion of
this risk taking tendency runs in families, (b) there is greater similarity between
siblings and their biological parents when it comes to risk taking than between
individuals and their adoptive parents, and (c) in matters of risk taking there is
more similarity between identical twins than between nonidentical twins. On the
basis of this and much more available data he predicts that: "In the future, as we

learn more, we're going to turn increasingly to the genes, the brain and the evolutionary story to understand ourselves—and not relentlessly insist that everything about us is attributable to something that happened either in school, in our relations with our parents or in some other aspect of environment and culture."[92]

Some additional evidence for a genetic predisposition to risk-taking comes from a study of compulsive gambling. It revealed that the spinal fluid and urine of chronic gamblers evidenced significantly higher levels of *norepinephrine*, a hormone that increases blood pressure, heart rate, and the rate and depth of breathing and is normally released under "fight or flight" conditions. Thus, gambling may supply the risk-taking behavior needed by a person with an abnormal secretion of this hormone. The researchers conclude that their findings support the "hypothesis that the personality trait of sensation-seeking may underlie risk-taking behavior, including pathological gambling, and that the biological substrata associated with sensation-seeking may be an increased tonic activity of the central noradrenergic system"[93] The study also revealed that more than 70 percent of the gambler subjects met the diagnostic criteria for severe depression and that there was a high incidence of depression and alcoholism in their families.

Scientists have long debated the relative proportions that biology and culture contribute to determining human behavior. This lengthy historical "nature versus nurture" controversy is not merely of academic interest, but has practical implications with respect to our survival potential. The relative contribution of genetics or environment, of course, will vary depending on the behavior in question. However, there is a growing recognition that an awareness of the biological underpinnings of certain life-shortening behaviors may help convince us to alter those behaviors before they take their final toll. Konner offers the example of alcohol abuse, which apparently has a strong biological component. In his view: "It is very important for people who carry that predisposition in their genes to be told that. It may mean that they have to monitor themselves more carefully or that they never take a drink. But if people don't start with the truth, it seems to me that they are in terrible trouble; they are carrying an unfair and unnecessary additional psychological burden as they go through life." Questions as to whether people in fact *prefer* to be told whether they have potentially harmful genes, or even if they *should* be told, raise important ethical implications. A surprising number of people simply don't want to know (or want others to know) the "truth" about the life-threatening components of their unique hereditary endowment.

The search for genetic and biological markers that might identify which individuals are most likely to develop cancer or heart disease has ushered in a new field called *molecular epidemiology*, also known as ecogenetics. Its practitioners seek to explain, among other things, the variations in how people respond to carcinogens. In this effort they are seeking to discover why, for instance, some heavy cigarette smokers get lung cancer while other heavy smokers do not, or why some employees succumb to workplace carcinogens while co-workers appear resistant to them. "The variations stem, ultimately, from the interaction between the environment and genes. The trick is to find signs of the interactions that raise or lower risk."[94]

Often such signs reflect genetic mutations of chromosones caused by carcinogens. An example is *aflatoxin*, which is a mold that grows on peanuts and corn. One gene, located on a specific chromosone, and "implicated in more than half of all cancers, becomes mutated in many liver cancer patients...in such a specific way that the change can be traced unambiguously to aflatoxin" (p.57). Hence, by screening people for the mutation one can identify those who have been harmed by aflatoxin, and they can be urged to seek early diagnosis and treatment. Treatment outcome will depend not only on their genetic makeup but also on their immune system, changes in dietary habits, subsequent exposure to carcinogens, and monitoring for early signs of tumors. Like many other promising life-saving developments discussed in this book, the findings from molecular epidemiology raise ethical quandries concerning such matters as mandatory versus voluntary screening, the rights of employers versus the rights of employees, protection against the potential misuse of genetic information, and issues of privacy and disclosure. Revelations from ecogenetics will no doubt provoke additional debate on these issues, as well as efforts to resolve them.

3

Risk-Taking Habits: Invitations to Death

The familiar saying that we are all "victims of habit" carries with it a great deal of truth. Indeed, social scientists have long recognized the importance of including habitual actions in developing theories of human conduct. Habitual activities can be defined as:

> ...stable response patterns that are learned through multiple repetitions until they become nearly or completely automatic responses to certain classes of stimuli. Some habits are learned via conscious mediation; but others are acquired without any awareness. Habits that are developed and perfected under conscious guidance often drop below the level of consciousness after they become over learned and well adjusted to environmental conditions. Well-learned habits are often performed so spontaneously and naturally that they may be spoken of as being "second nature"—in contrast to the biologically programmed responses that are "first nature."[95]

Habits, along with certain attitudes and related emotions, are part of the core of an individual's lifestyle. Many such routine behaviors also have some degree of risk taking associated with them. For some people, the chief threat to survival comes from life habits, repetitious behavior if you will, whose deleterious effects are known but are ignored.

In this Chapter, we look at some of the ways in which self-inflicted behaviors affect both the length and the quality of life. It's been estimated that perhaps half of all premature deaths (those that occur before the point of average longevity) can be related to lifestyle factors.[96] No more than 20 percent of these untimely deaths can be explained by heredity. Environmental factors (pollution, accidents, falls and the like) account for another 20 percent. Only 10 percent can be attributed to failures on the part of the medical-treatment system. Increasingly certain lifestyle factors are being identified as particularly crucial in the onset of a wide

31

range of chronic conditions and diseases. Analyses of heart disease provide an illustration of this connection. Researchers at Harvard Medical School sought to determine whether the long-term decline in ischemic heart disease was due to new medical or surgical interventions, changes in diet and lifestyle that are largely independent of the organized medical care system, or other factors.[97] An extensive review of the evidence led them to conclude that more than half of the decline in ischemic heart disease mortality was related to changes in lifestyle—specifically to reductions in serum cholesterol levels and smoking. Only 40 percent of the decline in mortality could be attributed to specific medical interventions, such as resuscitation efforts by coronary care units, medical treatment of ischemic heart disease, and the treatment of hypertension.

The Seven Deadly Sins.[98] That lifestyle factors can combine to affect health and longevity is further illustrated by a well known long term investigation that focused on the personal habits of 7,000 adults living in Alameda County, California.[99] It revealed that those who lived the longest followed most or all of seven practices: slept seven to eight hours a night, ate breakfast, rarely snacked between meals, maintained a reasonable weight, did not smoke, drank alcohol in moderation if at all, and took part in some sort of physical activity. Over a twelve year period the death rate for men adhering to all of these habits was only 28 percent that of men who observed only three or fewer. The comparable figure for women was 43 percent. Moreover, survival rates were substantially the same for those aged 65 and older as well as for those in younger age groups. The director of the study has noted: "The health habits one has at 65 are clearly related to one's subsequent mortality." In other words, even if these changes in lifestyle are not taken up until middle or later life, they still have the potential for improving health and, hopefully, extending life.[100]

A follow-up study further confirmed the self-destruction wrought by the seven unwholesome habits identified in the original Alameda County investigation.[101] The results clearly demonstrate that the more unhealthy habits people practiced, the greater their chances of dying prematurely. Moreover, poor health habits portend not only an early demise for many but chronic and costly disabilities for those who survive. That is to say, even when bad health habits do not lead to a premature death, they significantly increase the risk that an individual will suffer one or more physical or medical limitations that can seriously degrade the quality of life. In short, "preventive health practices are important not only in decreasing premature deaths but also in reducing costly debilitating illnesses."[102]

Habits: Installment Payments on Our Own Demise

Smoking, excessive eating, drug abuse, and alcoholism are all examples of a wide variety of habits which effectively reduce our life expectancies. In many instances these life-shortening habits reflect a person's direct involvement with his own *slow death*, which has been defined as "a predictable event, coming sooner rather than later, because of some systematic habit which threatens or injures health."[103] This process of death "on-the-installment-plan" refers to the fact that people cooperate in their own demise by continuing to engage in injurious patterns of behavior which they know have life-threatening consequences. Regardless of the flood of public warnings, they choose to disbelieve or ignore the fatal consequences of their own compulsive habits. Systematic inhalation of tobacco smoke, for instance, is like making potent, and often voluntary, installment payments toward an early annihilation.[104] In short, some personal habits can be deadly, and their continuation points toward a certain degree of culpability by millions of people in hastening their ultimate departure from this world. Some visible examples of how we help shape our own demise can be found by looking at two major causes of death in American society; that from cancer that begins with overexposure to the sun, and deaths resulting from auto accidents.

Skin Cancer. The most common form of cancer in the United States is skin cancer. The sun is responsible for 95 percent of all skin cancer, with well over one-half million cases reported annually. *Melanoma*, the most virulent and deadly form of skin cancer, also occurs through overexposure to ultraviolet rays. The lifetime incidence of melanoma has dramatically increased over the past several decades. Specifically, since 1930 the lifetime incidence of this form of skin cancer has gone from 1 in every 1500 people to 1 in every 150—a tenfold increase.[105] There has been a rapid worldwide increase in the melanoma rate, doubling with a concomitant rise in associated fatalities. In the United States thousands of new cases of melanoma are now being diagnosed each year and today thousands of citizens die from this form of cancer.

Other forms of skin cancer are serious, too. *Basal-cell carcinoma* now afflicts at least 400,000 Americans each year. This type of cancer usually appears on the face and other areas of the body which are exposed to the sun. Another common skin cancer is squamous-cell carcinoma. This type afflicts up to 100,000 Americans a year. These two types tend not to spread their cancer cells through the blood-stream as does melanoma. If they are ignored, however, they can be deadly. About 2,000 Americans die of these types of cancer a year. They can also cause disfigurement during the more advanced stages. It appears that skin cancers in general are developing at even younger ages, due to increased leisure time being spent outdoors. This should be a particular cause of concern, for there is evidence that youngsters who were severly sunburned at least once are twice as likely to develop melanoma in adulthood compared to those who had no such experience.

Despite the potential for fatal consequences, and the fact that most people are aware of the damaging effects of prolonged exposure to ultraviolet rays, millions continue to voluntarily bake their bodies under the sun, often merely to achieve a temporary but nevertheless "beautiful" tan. Moreover, many are not aware that several common drugs, for example, **tetracycline**, some diuretics, and even oral contraceptives, increase their sensitivity to the sun which, in turn, increases their risk of skin cancer through exposure.

Artificial tanning machines are similarly dangerous and risky. Most commercial tanning parlors use the UV-A wave-length band of ultraviolet light in their tanning booths. Scientists make the distinction between UV-A and UV-B wavelength bands. UV-A is the type which is the most dangerous and the most effective for tanning. This is the type of light which occurs around noon. The tanning parlors switched to UV-B in the belief that it is not harmful to the skin in the way that UV-A is. Scientists have found while UV-B itself seems to be harmless, in conjunction with UV-A it could be actually be worse for the skin than UV-A by itself.[106]

The knowledge and procedures necessary to minimize such risks are available. Avoiding overexposure in the first place is the first rule of survival. The proper use of a broad spectrum sunscreen is the second line of defense. Proper use means reapplication every few hours, as well as after swimming or perspiring heavily. A third essential precaution, especially if one is in the high risk group whose skin is especially susceptible to sunburn, is to have your body medically checked once a year. The American Academy of Dermatology has offered hundreds of screening programs across the United States in which participants learn how to examine themselves for signs of skin cancer.[107] With early detection, skin cancer is almost always curable. A treatment known as *chemosurgery* (also known as Mohs method or microscopic control surgery) apparently provides an almost 99 percent chance for cure *if* the affliction is caught in time.[108]

Minimizing the risks associated with achieving a temporary bronze complexion that can only be maintained through more hours under the sun or another trip to the tanning salon is not difficult. Avoiding overexposure, properly using sun screen products, and annual medical examinations are usually sufficient steps to reduce the risk of contracting severe cases of melanoma. The importance of these behavioral modifications becomes especially apparent as one ages. Malignant melanoma is a deceptive disease because it requires 30 to 40 years of exposure to manifest its effects. In a case such as this, where the benefits of preventive measures are long term, corrective action at the moment often appears unnecessary to many sunbathers. However, they would do well to change their attitude and to institute a more guarded approach to sunbathing and to heed the dramatic warning of the American Cancer Society, succinctly summed up in their message: "Fry now, pay later." Or, as one writer similarly put it: "Getting blistering sunburn today may be signing your own death warrant for tomorrow." Dermatologic research is making great advances in the molecular biology and immunology of skin cancer, but to date, the best protection against dangerous burns comes from the exercise of individual precaution to minimize the risks. It may just prolong your survival time.

Why Don't We Buckle Up?

Just as one can take precaution against skin cancer becoming a threat to life, so one can significantly reduce the risk of injury from accidents. A significant proportion are due to motor vehicle crashes alone. At least 40,000 Americans die each year, and thousands of others are severely injured as well, as a result of motor vehicle crashes. What is interesting here is that the technology to prevent the vast majority of these fatalities and injuries is the car seat belt. However, various polls show that only a minority of Americans report that they *always* wear seat belts. This is discouraging, since without this precaution, a person is twice as likely to be killed or seriously injured in an accident. Studies show that in an accident where seat belts are not used, the front-seat passenger is 2 1/2 times more likely to be killed, and the driver is four times more likely to die than a person who is buckled in.

Traffic safety expert agree that if drivers would simply "buckle up" before starting their engines, the probability of car deaths would be significantly reduced. However, it has been estimated that while compliance is rising, only a minority of the driving population consistently utilizes seat belts on a regular basis. The National Highway Traffic Safety Administration claims that regular usage would reduce traffic deaths by at least 14,500 a year.[109]

Why significant numbers of people fail to take this simple, but voluntary, precaution—and thereby increase their survival potential—remains something of a mystery. There are, no doubt, a variety of reasons, including laziness and the false sense that one will be able to react in time to avoid serious injury or death. This would indicate that they generally don't understand the physical forces operative in an automobile accident. A vivid description of those forces is provided in the following description of a person driving 40 miles per hour that crashes into a fixed object:

> Immediately on impact, my body is hurtling toward the dashboard at almost 60 feet per second. I can't stop myself with my hands—that would be like bench-pressing at least 3500 pounds. Inevitably, my stomach rams the steering wheel. Meanwhile, my legs instinctively stiffen and crack at the knees. My right knee wedges under the dash. As the firewall buckles upward, the leg snaps just above the ankle. My upper legs, jammed into the dash, resist the forward motion of my torso, dislocating my hip joints instantly. My upper body is jackknifing forward. Less than a tenth of a second into the crash, it slams into the steering column. My breastbone caves in just before my ribs start to break. Little room remains in my chest for my lungs, heart and aorta, while the broken bones have become spears. Now my head is smashing into the windshield, crushing my nose and cheekbones. It strikes at the same speed I would attain by diving into the sidewalk from a second-story window. My brain simultaneously slams into my forehead and rips away from the back of my skull. Then it rebounds, crushing and ripping again.[110]

The National Highway Traffic Safety Administration has noted some of the more common reasons that people give for not wearing safety belts and how each of them are not supported by the facts. For example: (a) "Seat belts are only necessary on long trips or in bad weather." The truth is that most accidents occur within 25 miles of home, during good weather, and on dry pavement. (b) "I can't drive all strapped in like that. Seat belts are too confining." New safety belt technology allow the wearer freedom of movement to operate all the controls in an automobile. A special locking mechanism only engages when the car stops suddenly. (c) "I'd rather be thrown clear of the accident." This would be fine if you could choose where you would land; however, you're likely to be thrown onto concrete or into the path of oncoming traffic. Being thrown from the car makes you 25 times more likely to suffer a fatal injury during a crash. (d) "I don't want to be trapped inside a car that is burning or is submerged in water." Being tossed about without a safety belt might knock you unconscious or otherwise injure you, making it impossible for you to escape. Crashes involving fire or submersion account for less than one half of one percent of all automobile crashes.

Whatever the reasons, seat belt installation in automobiles has failed to achieve its maximum potential for reducing the risk of premature mortality. It is true that the past few years has witnessed a decline in mortality from car accidents. However, traffic safety experts attribute this decline to mandatory lower speed limits, the rise in the minimum drinking age in several states, and to intensified police efforts to combat driving by those who are alcohol-impaired. People are still in the negative habit of not taking the simple forethought to "buckle up." The Highway Users Federation, a group that supports mandatory seat belt use laws, estimates that if 80 percent of people in cars wore seat belts, the country could save over $5 billion a year on accident-related medical bills, legal expenses and other costs. Others have put this figure as high as $6 billion.

Mandatory seat belt usage bills have been introduced and intensely debated in various legislatures across the country. In 1984, New York became the first state to pass such a law and, as of that year, about 30 countries had mandatory-use laws. Studies showed that in most of these countries, belt use doubled or tripled immediately after the law went into effect. It then tends to drop off, later rising again to a plateau. In that same year the U.S. Department of Transportation issued a ruling making air bags, or some other form of passive restraint system, mandatory of all cars sold in the U. S. by 1990. Beginning with the 1990 models, automobile manufacturers were required to equip all passenger cars with automatic crash protection devices. Today all cars are equipped with either safety belts or air bag systems or both. Experts point out, however, that although seat belt laws are effective in the short-run, they may not be effective in the long-run. For example, in January of one year, nearly 70 percent of all New Yorkers buckled up, but by September, less than 50 percent were using seat belts.[111] In other words, over time complacency sets in and people revert to earlier careless habits of driving.

There is also a problem in that most of the new seat belt laws are limited to enforcement *only* when the driver of the car is stopped for another traffic violation. For such laws to be truly effective the police must have the authority to stop cars in which the occupants aren't using seat belts, whether they are breaking any other rules or not. It boils down to a major problem of inadequate enforcement with minimal fines.[112]

Cell Phones: The New Hazard. The widespread adoption of cell phone technology has introduced new hazards on the road. They have become a major driver distraction and are responsible for a growing number of accidents. Some communities are beginning to ban their use while driving. Unfortunately, many choose to ignore the law, needlessly putting their lives and those of others at risk.

There are countless individuals who choose to take on such risks or resist the utilization of "passive restraints" (air bags that inflate automatically in a crash, or automatic seat belts that wrap around occupants as car doors close). In the past, automobile and insurance industries, as well as politicians, often wasted considerable time contesting and debating issues surrounding occupant protection systems while people were being mutilated and killed on the streets and highways. That resistance declined as the life-saving and economic value of such systems gained increasing appreciation.

Many find the laws requiring restraints intrusive and a violation of their rights as individuals. One can only view as perverse the notion that one has the freedom to place the lives of others in jeopardy. As Imperato and Mitchell have noted, "the problem with so-called "voluntary" risks…is that one person's chosen risk has a way of becoming another person's imposed risk—as thousands of victims of drunk driving find out every year"(xii). The fact of the matter is that people won't always buckle up unless it's the law—*and* that law is strictly enforced with swift and consistent punishment of all violators. Until that happens, we can look forward to the continuation of thousands of unnecessary deaths and injuries each year from risks we take behind the wheel of an automobile.

4

Lifestyle Habits: Invitations to Live

Physical Exercise: A Life-Saving Enhancer

A major theme throughout this book is that individuals can develop their approach to daily living in a variety of ways so as to improve their health and survival potential. One obvious and well-known enhancing activity is exercise. Not only does a regimen of proper exercise help one physically *and* psychologically, such activity is also life-saving—it lengthens life and reduces the risk of heart disease and stroke.[113] In fact, regular physical exertion can greatly reduce the risks of a variety of diseases and conditions, including hypertension, diabetes, osteoporosis, obesity, stress, depression, and anxiety.[114] It has also been associated with a lower rate of colon cancer and reduced back injury.[115] Given the preponderance of beneficial evidence, one can argue that people who do not regularly exercise are failing to take advantage of a relatively cost-free and proven means to prevent premature mortality.

Despite the multiplicity of potential health benefits, it appears that only a minority of adults exercise on a regular basis. The U.S. Department of Health and Human Services reports that the large majority of Americans lead too sedentary a lifestyle. This is of considerable concern, since an inactive lifestyle appears to be an independent risk factor associated with coronary heart disease, nearly doubling an individual's vulnerability. A long-term study of high-risk men by the National Institute of Health found that those who engaged in at least 30 minutes of moderate physical exercise each day had one-third fewer fatal heart attacks than those who did less than a half hour a day. Sufficient exercise was defined as anything which raises heart and lung performance to 60 percent of their capacity for twenty minutes, three times a week. However, most people even when they do exercise do not do so in a manner to achieve maximum cardiovascular benefits. Nevertheless, even mild forms of activity like raking leaves, walking up stairs, golfing, light sports, house and yard work, and so on can be mentally and physically rewarding. In other words, some pattern of habitual movement, even such things as increasing your standing and stretching moments over sitting time, can contribute to overall fitness and a feeling of well-being.[116]

While the public has generally been made aware of the importance of physical fitness, only a minority has taken the required course of action. Indeed, we are not in so good a shape as we might think. Government reports show that slightly over a fifth of all adults engage in at least 30 minutes of light to moderate physical activity 5 or more times per week. Only 10 percent of the population exercises vigorously and regularly enough (3 or more times a week) to improve their cardio-respiratory fitness. A significant number of adults report no leisure-time physical activity, and the prevalence of such sedentary behavior increases with age. This is discouraging, since the latest medical knowledge clearly shows that moderate physical exercise can be helpful in countering the effects of previous negative lifestyle habits, even at older ages.

Exercise and Aging. Among the elderly exercise can increase functional status and thereby extend independent living. It can have a beneficial impact on certain chronic diseases prevalent among persons 65 years of age and older. Of the four most common chronic diseases found among this group—arthritis, hypertension, hearing impairment, and heart disease—three are known to positively respond to regular physical activity. Exercise can help control weight, blood pressure, and blood sugar, and improve flexibility and range of motion among those who have arthritis. Physical activity and exercise are factors that contribute to increased life expectancy among the elderly. This was the case in a longitudinal study of a national sample of persons who were at least 70 years of age. Analysis revealed that there was a higher number of deaths among older persons who reported lower activity or exercise levels. Self-assessments of four activities—being less active than peers, not getting enough exercise, not having a regular exercise routine, and walking a mile less than once a week—were all significantly associated with mortality. The same variables also predicted mortality among women. These findings tend to confirm the importance to older persons of maintaining voluntary activity in their life styles.[117]

Unfortunately, too few older Americans are getting even moderate amounts of exercise. As so often is the case in other domains of living, socioeconomic conditions play a role—the old-old, women, and low-income, less educated populations are least likely to exercise regularly. Older adults may also avoid regular physical activity for a variety of other reasons:

They may be unaware of the potential benefits. They may have misconceptions about exercise. The chronic illnesses common to this population may make older adults feel they are unable to exercise. Then too, the older generation, especially older women, have had little experience with sports and other forms of physical activity. Yet others, such as those who have worked at manual labor during their lifetimes, may feel they should rest once retired. The presence of younger, more "fit" participants in general programs may be intimidating or physically or socially uncomfortable for the older adult.[118]

Whatever the reasons, much more needs to be done to inform as well as convince the older generation of the positive advantages of regular physical activity.

Creative programs that encourage participation, such as low-impact aerobic dancing or muscle strengthening sessions, can improve the physical conditioning of members of this large and relatively sedentary group. Although the image of the young, oiled, muscle-bound body builders has been with us for a long time, we are only just beginning to appreciate the health benefits of moderate muscle building workouts for the general population, including the very old. Much can be done to counter the muscle atrophy that results from lack of physical activity. In one experiment, some nursing home patients ranging in age from 86 to 96, most of who suffered from arthritis, heart disease, and high blood pressure, were placed on a weight training program designed to strengthen their legs. After only two months, the participants had doubled, tripled and quadrupled their leg strength. A few were even able to discard their walking canes. Many were still gaining in strength at the program's end. Mild exercise has even been shown to strengthen the bones of women in their 80s. While we cannot stop the aging process, "good eating habits coupled with regular aerobic and resistance exercise can help delay or prevent the so-called declining years. If we must go gentle into that good night, at least we'll be able to carry our own luggage."[119]

A Sedentary Nation. Despite all the joggers visible on the streets and in the parks, it appears that the impression of an exercise momentum among our citizenry is somewhat illusory. For example, a Gallup Leisure Audit found little change in the number of sports participants in the preceding two years. Indeed, at the time of the survey a little under one third of the men and over one-third of the women were obese. These were about the same proportions found a decade earlier. The director of the Adult Behavioral Risk Factor Surveillance Survey for the Federal Centers for Disease Control and Prevention similarly noted that the small percentage of Americans who were physically active is about the same as it was a decade earlier. He pointed out that nearly three out of five adults in America lead sedentary lives, spending less than three 20-minute sessions a week, that is, one-hour a week, at leisure-time physical activity. Hence, he characterizes the notion that Americans are becoming more active as simply a myth.[120]

The poorer segments of our population, and children, are particularly inactive when it comes to leisure-time physical exercise. The poor cannot afford such things like private tennis lessons, swimming and skating lessons, and member-ships in health clubs or even the local YMCA. The highest shares of sedentary adults are found in areas with large low-income populations. For example, in the District of Columbia, home of the nation's capital, over 73 percent of adults are sedentary, and nearly 52 percent get no physical activity at all. Such figures are cause for concern, given that: "Lack of physical activity is the most prevalent behavioral risk factor for heart disease in this country, far surpassing smoking and obesity."[121]

Thus, most people have not done what is required to stay in shape, that is, build regular physical activity into their daily lives as part of a permanent lifestyle. It takes a certain degree of stick-to-itiveness to adhere to this habit of living. It is not easy. Apparently only a small minority of persons, perhaps 10 percent, can maintain the necessary motivation to exercise consistently. A similar percentage stubbornly refuses to alter its sedentary ways. There is data showing that nearly 29 percent of all adults in the nation get no exercise whatsoever. Some have char-acterized them as the "incorrigibly immobile." The vast majority of people fitfully tries, in varying ways and degrees, to improve their health habits, but is not very successful.[122] Often, after a relapse or two, the inclination is to give up.

At the same time many continue to hope to find an easier way, a shortcut to good health. Some get caught up in a roller-coaster pattern of dieting. They adopt first one and then another of the latest diet fads promoted through the mass media, hoping to find a fast and effortless way to get their bodies in shape. An ubiquitous army of quacks promising quick fixes stands ever ready to promise instant miracles, like the "lose weight while you sleep" pill recently advertised in newspapers across the country. It states in part:

> ...the pill itself does all the work while you quickly lose weight with NO star-vation 'diet menus' to follow, NO exercise and NO hunger pangs...One beautiful thing about these miracle pills is the ease with which they work. The best time to take the pills is just before you go to bed at night. That way, the pounds melt away even as you sleep. You wake up every morning, slimmer, happier, and feeling younger.

Imagine—achieving the fountain of youth while you are asleep! However, as Salisbury reminds us: "there is no shortcut to life. To the end of our days, life is a lesson imperfectly learned."[123]

And the lesson, though imperfectly learned, is simple: physical activity is an important form of risk intervention. A regular regimen of walking, for example, renders positive feedback to the person through a feeling of control over his or her personal responsibility and commitment to remaining healthy. This one activity often tends to motivate the participant to become further involved in other related interventions such as attending to cholesterol and caloric intakes, instituting weight-control measures, and monitoring blood pressure. Research has shown that brisk walking every day leads to weight loss and reduces the risks of heart disease. Exercise of this nature, to be beneficial, does not necessarily require a pattern of persistent overexertion. A study of Harvard alumni (all male and primarily white), for example, found that those who engaged in such moderate exercise as walking and climbing stairs live up to two years longer than their more sedentary peers. Moreover, it was found that a lifetime habit of engaging in energetic activity three to four times a week could reduce the negative health consequences of smoking or high blood pressure. It can even partly offset an inherited tendency toward early death.[124]

Numerous investigations have confirmed the life-saving and life-extending benefits of exercise.[125] For instance, the Lifestyle Heart Trial, conducted at the University of California, demonstrated that it was sometimes possible to undo serious coronary disease damage after one year of a changed lifestyle. Patients during this period who exercised more frequently and longer, and consumed fewer calories and less cholesterol, experienced an overall regression in coronary atherosclerosis comparable to that achieved through drug therapy. In a control group that did not change its lifestyle, the atherosclerosis condition worsened. In short, a program of regular exercise, carried out on a moderate scale, can reduce the risk of premature death, improve the quality of living, and at the same time prolong life. The well known maxim "use it or lose it" may be a cogent shorthand for a real truth. The commitment to exercise must be a lifetime proposition.[126]

The Perils of Smoking

By now the vast majority of people are aware of the potentially lethal consequences of smoking. Indeed, one of the most remarkable cultural shifts in attitudes that has taken place in the past decade has been from a general societal approval of this life-threatening habit to one of widespread disapproval. Smokers now complain of the public and private restrictions increasingly imposed on them in terms of where they can engage in this behavior. Volatile emotional and sometimes physical encounters between those who do and those who do not smoke are reported in the press and popular weekly magazines as pressures mount to curtail, if not eliminate, the practice. Arguments erupt over whether smoking is a constitutional right protected along with other individual freedoms or whether it is a privilege which can be limited or denied. Offices, sometimes entire buildings, now often have "No Smoking" placards posted; restaurants are commonly divided into smoking and nonsmoking sections, cigarette manufacturers are required to place health warnings on their products; and airlines now prohibit passenger smoking. The practice is increasingly prohibited on public conveyances, elevators, and other public space, etc. The author knows of one person who had a sign prominently displayed on her front door which said: "Absolutely No Smoking Allowed in This Home!" Moreover, someone attempting to light up in her car will be quickly admonished to end that "filthy habit" then and there! While this may sound extreme, it is more likely indicative of a growing aggressiveness on the part of the non-smoking public toward the still rather large population of people who use tobacco.

Despite this shift in emphasis and a growing intolerance of those who refuse to quit, significant numbers of people still puff away on cigarettes, cigars, or pipes. Tobacco use is the most important single preventable cause of death and disease in American society. However, like so many habits, smoking can become an addictive behavior pattern and, when it does, it becomes extremely difficult to give it up, even for those who are most acutely aware of its consequences. For example, "virtually all physicians know of colleagues—even chest surgeons—who remain so greatly addicted that they are unable to discontinue smoking despite the presence of serious, progressive tobacco-related illness."[127] Physicians who are tobacco dependent are, of course, only a small part of a much larger army of people who have experienced unsuccessful efforts to "shake the habit" even in the face of the broad spectrum of illnesses and fatal diseases it provokes.

Cigarette smoking has noticeably declined in this country since the first Surgeon General's report on its effects appeared in 1964. Nevertheless, it remains a major risk factor for millions of people, smokers and non-smokers alike, causing unnecessary and life-threatening illnesses. Tobacco is a major risk factor for diseases of the heart and blood vessels; chronic bronchitis and emphysema; cancers of the lung, larynx, oral cavity, esophagus, pancreas, and bladder; and other problems such as respiratory infections and stomach ulcers.

Other People's Smoke. The Environmental Protection Agency estimates that thousands of *nonsmokers* die each year from lung cancer caused by inhaling other people's tobacco smoke. So-called "side stream smoke" emitted into the air from a smoldering cigarette sometimes includes carcinogens in higher concentrations than those inhaled directly by the smoker. Nonsmoking women married to smoking men may find themselves in particularly hazardous circumstances. Children are about twice as likely to take up the habit if either parent has already done so. Moreover, so-called "secondhand smoke" is especially dangerous. Evidence from studies cited in the Surgeon General reports reveals that children in smoking households have an increased incidence of respiratory symptoms and occurrence of bronchitis and pneumonia. In addition, they miss more days of school and experience more frequent hospitalizations.[128]

As the decade of the 1990's began, tobacco use was responsible for more than one of every six deaths in the United States. The overall death rate for cigarette smokers is 70 percent higher than for nonsmokers. As of this writing, cigarette smoking alone accounted for over 390,000 premature deaths per year, including more than 20 percent of all coronary heart disease deaths, nearly 90 percent of lung cancer deaths, and 30 percent of all cancer deaths. Even though cigarette smoking is the largest preventable cause of premature death and illness, nearly one-third of all adults in 1990 still manifested the nicotine habit. Yet the majority of them knew this was a major risk factor for heart disease.

Tobacco and Alcohol: A Dangerous Mix. Cigarette smoking interacts with alcohol to increase the onset of cancer of the oral cavity, esophagus, and larynx. The reason for this deadly mix is that the two substances interact in a *synergistic* fashion, that is, in combination they make each other more powerful and hence cause more damage than either would do alone. Therefore, simultaneous exposure to tobacco and alcohol invites a greater risk from this "double jeopardy" of developing upper respiratory illnesses as well as cardiovascular diseases.[129]

Smoking also has adverse effects for pregnant women and those using oral contraceptives. Their babies tend to be smaller at birth and more vulnerable to disease during their first year. Moreover, maternal smoking may be detrimental to a child's long-term physical and intellectual development. It should come as no surprise to learn that smoking rates remain the highest among certain populations associated with lower socioeconomic status—blacks, blue-collar workers, people with lower educational levels, and so on.

The idea that reduced tar and nicotine levels in cigarettes will help alleviate the effects of smoking remains questionable. People apparently compensate for the reduction by either smoking more, inhaling more deeply, or puffing more frequently in order to get the same satisfying level of nicotine. In any event, low-tar-and-nicotine cigarettes are no replacement for the difficult but necessary choice of abstention. In addition, increased prohibitions against smoking in public places lessen the risk that nonsmokers will develop maladies associate with smoking.[130] Despite such incidents, one might be wise to remember that each time a person lights up he or she is making another voluntary installment payment on their own demise.[131]

It's Never Too Late To Quit

It has long been known that most smokers in fact want to quit. The majority, when questioned, voice regret over having started in the first place. However, it is not an easy habit to abandon, although many try. Within a year of quitting, four-fifths will light up again. Only between 20 and 30 percent are successful in quitting permanently. Why? Nonsmokers often do not understand why this habit has such a powerful hold on people or why so many take it up again after a period of abstinence, given what is now known about its hazards. The reasons smokers stay "hooked" are many and complex. A major inducement is to avoid the anguish of the nicotine withdrawal process. There also are powerful psychopharmacological benefits which people feel help them to cope with the vicissitudes of life. Researchers report nicotine produces temporary improvements in behavior and mood. For example, it makes it easier to perform daily tasks, relieves anxiety ("It relaxes me."), improves memory ("It helped me to think and concentrate"), reduces hunger and increases tolerance of pain. Smoking provides may people with a sense of pleasure and well-being. "Smoking can soothe or stimulate, focus the mind or serve as a social prop. More crucially, the desire for a cigarette is reinforced by daily rituals or social situations: every cup of coffee, every cocktail, every meeting or waiting room presents a challenge."[132] Despite the short-term benefits, the long-term consequences of smoking in terms of its deleterious effect on our health and longevity can hardly be ignored.

On the positive side, evidence is mounting that no matter how long one has been a smoker, quitting provides beneficial effects. For example, a national Coronary Artery Surgery Study revealed that those 65 and older and at risk for coronary artery disease who quit smoking reduced their chances of experiencing a heart attack or early death just as much as quitters who were aged 35 to 55. Even among those who have been smoking for decades can partially reverse its effects within one to five years after quitting.[133] Evidence from the Surgeon General reports indicate that quitting "cold turkey" may be a more effective strategy than gradually reducing consumption without attempting to stop entirely. Indeed, the vast majority, perhaps over 95 percent, of those who do manage to break the habit do so without the help of organized programs.

Women: The New Risk Takers

While the proportion of smokers has been declining, that downward trend has been noticeably slower among women. Moreover, among some female age-groups, smoking may in fact be increasing. In a very real sense, they have become the new risk takers.[134] Today nearly one in three women of reproductive age are smokers, often not recognizing that such behavior may have adverse affects on their fertility, pregnancy, and the well-being of the child. Smoking during pregnancy increases the risk of miscarriage, premature birth, lower infant birth weight, and sudden infant death syndrome. Moreover, if women smoke while using oral contraceptives, they run a greater risk of heart attack, which generally is rare in younger women. The report by the Center for Disease Control, referred to earlier, showed that over two-fifths of white women aged 18 to 24 were smokers, and that half of them were also taking birth control pills, a potentially hazardous combination of substances.

The increased rates of smoking behavior among young women can in part be attributed to the realization of certain values such as individualism, freedom, and equality, long associated with the women's suffrage movement. Greater access to education, jobs, and political power has given many women an opportunity to assert their own individuality. Cigarette smoking appears to be associated with these trends. Nor has this been an unanticipated revolution. Tobacco companies have long actively marketed certain cigarette brands aimed specifically at the younger, female consumer. During the eighties, for example, two-page advertisements for the Virginia Slims brand, picturing pretty women with cigarettes in their hands and touting the message "You've come a long way, baby," were common. They played to the growing emancipation of women by portraying cigarette smoking as a symbol of their greater freedom and equality, especially in comparison to women of the past. The opposite page of this particular advertisement would portray women of the past comparatively drab both in looks and in dress. Those seduced by the slick advertisement could look forward to paying a heavy price. For example, women who are heavy smokers are more than six times as likely to suffer a stroke as nonsmokers. Even light smokers have over twice the risk of stroke than those who have never smoked.[135] Lung cancer has risen dramatically in women over the last few decades, reflecting partly that aging population of women who started smoking after World War II and now are evidencing the consequences of having done so. It now surpasses breast cancer as the number one killer of women.

The Double Standard: Look Slim and Young. One of the major reasons women offer for their inability to stop smoking or for relapsing after quitting is a fear of gaining weight. The potential for adding pounds is real; a majority of ex-smokers do put on weight, at least initially, with women getting heavier than men. In a sense, the female suffers from a double standard of aging. Cultural expectations pressure her to remain slim and young looking while men are allowed to age with "character," regardless of a protruding paunch and other signs of physical decline. The fear of not being able to meet these cultural expectations, irrational as they may be, prevent at least some women from kicking the habit, that is, they elect to keep on smoking in order to avoid putting on extra poundage. This is obviously a stressful no-win situation and contributes to what analysts refer to as the *living-dangerously syndrome*: compared to nonsmokers, smokers tend to drink more, sleep less, exercise less, skip breakfast, use seat belts less, use drugs and medication more often, and have a greater tendency to carry guns or knives. People exhibiting this syndrome are clearly compounding risks and stacking the odds in favor of an early demise.

It is well known that the earlier one begins smoking, the more difficult it is to stop. While there is some variation from survey to survey, estimates of prevalence of smoking among teenagers have been as high as 36 percent. National surveys also reveal that despite the fact that the vast majority of teenagers have been exposed to information related to the health risks of smoking, nevertheless for many the perceived benefits of smoking outweighed the risks involved.[136] Toward the end of the 1980's it appeared that tobacco companies had begun anew to target their advertisements toward a large population of persons known for their propensity to risk taking, namely, young and impressionable adolescents. The companies generally deny any such intent. However, several studies showed that the promotional efforts of one marketer, designed around a hip-looking cartoon mascot named Joe Camel, were extremely effective in attracting teenage smokers to its product.[137] How effective? The researchers estimate that Camel sales to youngsters rose from $6 million a year prior to the Joe Camel ad campaign to $476 million in 1991.

Related evidence of a focus on adolescent smokers comes from their use of so-called smokeless tobacco, namely, snuff. Reports from the American Academy of Otolaryngology—Head and Neck Surgery, indicate that while cigarette sales declined 18 percent in one decade, moist snuff, the only form of tobacco posting a sales gain, experienced a 50 percent increase. According to the U.S. Department of Health and Human Services, long-term users are up to 50 times more likely to develop cancers of the cheek and gum than people who don't use snuff. An estimated 12 million people—a fourth of whom is under 21 years of age—use smokeless tobacco. Boys as young as 8 mimic snuff-using baseball heroes only to have problems later. Of teenage users, more than half develop mouth sores after an average of only 3.3. years of use.

Unfortunately, the adult role models exhibit increased vulnerability to disease and death. In a study of over one-thousand baseball players, 38 percent reported current smokeless tobacco use. Slightly more than 46 percent of these users had *oral leukoplakia*—leathery white or red patches inside the mouth that can become cancerous, compared to only 1.4 percent of the non-users. Smokeless tobacco may also increase the risk of heart disease. HDL cholesterol blood levels appear to drop as **cotinine**, a byproduct of nicotine, levels rise. Decreased HDL levels are associated with increased risk of heart disease. And, if this isn't enough, the use of snuff is also associated with bad breath, tooth decay, permanently stained teeth, gum recession leading to tooth loss, decreased sense of taste and smell, increased heart rate, constricted blood vessels and high blood pressure![138]

The power of the advertising industry is worth noting. It has been found that magazines which rely heavily on cigarette advertising are far less likely than others to includes articles on the dangers of smoking. In an analysis of nearly 100 magazines published over the past 25 years, it was demonstrated that magazines carrying tobacco ads were 38 percent less likely to discuss smoking risks than those without such ads. In short, there was a strong link between increasing ad spending and declining coverage: as cigarette ad revenues increased, the magazines' likelihood of covering smoking risks decreased. This was especially true, surprisingly, for women's magazines: they were 50 percent less likely to cover the health dangers of smoking than other women's magazines that didn't run the ads. Apparently, those publications with significant revenues from tobacco industry advertisements appear to engage in a form of self-censorship in order not to offend a major source of income.[139] In the words of one executive editor, magazines are reluctant "to bite the hand that feeds them."[140] It has been argued that such self-censorship may lead to gross under-estimation of the importance of smoking and health on the part of the average person.

While the sale of tobacco has declined in this country in recent years, the industry has compensated for that trend in two ways—promoting discount cigarettes and so-called private-label brands, and selling its products in other parts of the world.

Discount Cigarettes. A report from the United States Surgeon General stated that every 10 percent rise in the price of cigarettes leads to a 4 percent decline in smoking. However, the surge in discount sales has disrupted that connection, and has interrupted the steady decline in cigarette consumption. Keeping the price affordable has enticed thousands of people who might have quit to switch to cheaper cigarettes in order to continue the habit.[141]

Exporting the Habit. It has been estimated that cigarette and raw tobacco sales overseas have dramatically increased over the years.[142] The shipping of potentially life-threatening products as well as environmental contaminants, often to other third-world countries, is not an uncommon practice. In many instances, the regulatory mechanisms in those countries are ineffective in monitoring the importation of such products and assessing their health consequences. Toward the end of the first Bush administration, pressure was being exerted on South Korea, Thailand, Japan, and other nations to open their markets to tobacco products, despite strong protests of anti-smoking organizations such as the American Medical Association and the American Cancer Society. As one editorial put it, "They send us televisions, automobiles and VCRs—and we send them packs of lingering death."

Making Smoking Costly. Several countries have discovered that the imposition of heavy cigarette taxes can dramatically change a personal habit that unnecessarily burdens public health budgets already suffering from soaring medical costs and growing demands for hospital care. Studies completed in several industrial countries reveal that raising the price of cigarettes is an effective way to reduce smoking, especially among teenagers. Using taxes in this instance to shape public behavior is seen as making sound fiscal sense. "With public health care costs already overwhelming government budgets, cigarette taxes offer an extraordinary opportunity for politicians: a way to cut public costs without cutting pubic services—and at the same time to raise new revenues without raising hell with the electorate."[143]

Alcohol Misuse

Approximately one out of ten deaths in this country are related to alcohol. The misuse of alcohol leads to death from disease and accidents. For example, data from the International Agency for Research on Cancer shows that persons who both smoke and drink heavily are 44 times more likely to suffer from cancer of the esophagus than nonsmokers.[144] Accidents, especially those involving motor vehicles, also often take the lives of others besides the driver. Drunk driving kills thousands Americans each year, and injures more than a half-million. Alcohol has been implicated in almost half of all deaths caused by motor vehicle crashes and fatal intentional injuries, such as suicides and homicides. Some may be surprised to learn that victims are intoxicated in about one-third of all suicides, drownings, and beating deaths.[145]

Estimates of the dollar costs to business and industry from alcoholic problems range from $50 billion to well over a $100 billion a year. The majority of such costs are attributed to lost employment and reduced productivity. Ten million on-the-job accidents a year are alcohol related, two million of them disabling. Alcoholics use a disproportionate share of our health resources. Health care costs for untreated alcoholics have been found to be at least 100 percent higher than those for nonalcoholic.

The Female Drinker and Breast Cancer

As was the case with smoking, women are increasingly at risk with respect to alcoholic consumption. We have already noted the dangerous synergistic effect of tobacco and alcohol, which accelerates the carcinogenic process, thereby increasing the probabilities of cancer of the throat, larynx, and esophagus. Women who smoke heavily and drink are apt to develop cancers of the oral cavity and tongue at younger ages. Early studies had also suggested an alcohol/breast cancer connection. However, most of these early results were obtained *retrospectively*, that is, women were first queried about their drinking habits and then their responses were compared with women without the disease. The problem with retrospective information is that if a woman knows that she has breast cancer, that might color her recollection and distort description of past behavior. Two more recent *prospective* studies, in which women were first asked about their lifestyles, and then followed over time, corrects this problem. Both studies revealed that women who drank had a higher probability of developing breast cancer. As might be expected, the risk of breast cancer increased with the amount of alcohol consumed. Drinking seems to pose the greatest hazard for younger women.[146],[147]

The number of women afflicted with breast cancer has risen. Some of this increase is due to better detection efforts, but a significant proportion reflects a higher rate. Nearly all of this increase occurred in women over 50 years old. Two decades ago only one in twenty women got breast cancer. Today, the figure is one in nine. Little progress has been made in reducing the death rate from this disease. During this twenty-year period the percentage of women who died from it has remained virtually the same (about 45,000 a year), despite advances in medical treatment, and wider use of *mammography*, and more accurate detection of tumors in their early stages of development.

We still lack the fundamental knowledge about the causes and growth of breast cancer. There are certain statistical associations which are not quite understood, For example, a woman whose mother had breast cancer has a risk three to four times greater than a female without a family history of cancer. Women whose menopause starts at age 55 or later have twice the risk of those whose menopause begins prior to age 50. In recent years medical researchers have focused their attention on the role that diet plays, especially the role of fat consumption. There already is general agreement that the levels of fat in Western diets are perilously high and can lead to various chronic diseases such as colon cancer and heart disease. Now some medical researchers suggest that fat-laden diets may explain the high rates of breast cancer in the United States and other wealthy nations. For example, in Japan, the consumption of fast foods (hamburgers, pizzas, etc.) has made inroads into the traditional diet of fish, rice, and vegetables. This shift in eating habits has been accompanied by a concomitant rise in breast cancer."[148]

Much more needs to be known about these and other factors associated with breast cancer. In the meantime, women can initiate several strategies to minimize their vulnerability to this disease. We have already noted in this connection the adverse effects of tobacco and alcohol consumption. Conclusive or unequivocable scientific proof linking fat intake and breast cancer is still being sought. Nevertheless, the available evidence suggests that reducing the amount of fat in one's diet may also lessen a woman's risk of developing breast cancer. As Misch notes, "the prudent thing to do, as with trying to avoid heart disease by not smoking, would be to treat fatty foods as a delicacy you allow yourself only every once in awhile." (p. 36) Early detection is essential, since tumors are more treatable in the early stages of development, and can improve chances of survival dramatically. This means getting regular breast exams. Unfortunately, more than half of the women over the age of 40 have never had a mammogram, thereby placing themselves at greater risk. One apparent reason for this is the lack of health insurance. A significant proportion of the 45 million or so Americans currently without health coverage are women.[149] As is so often the case, people without adequate insurance coverage receive fewer benefits and poorer care than those with private health insurance. For example, in one survey of nearly 100 hospitals in Illinois, it was found that breast-cancer patients at urban hospitals were more likely to receive a diagnosis late in the disease, and were less likely to receive radiation therapy, than patients treated at more affluent facilities.[150]

We have previously stressed the importance of pregnant women recognizing the dangerous combined effects of tobacco and alcohol, especially as they impact on the long-term development of the child. Given such outcomes, it is dismaying to learn from the University of North Carolina Highway Safety Research Center that during a eight-year period, although the number of men arrested in that state for driving while intoxicated DWI) declined by 9 percent, the number of women arrested for a similar offense rose by 43 percent. Again, this may be a reflection of the growing emancipation of women, as well as a shift in attitudes and values. Some hypothesize that the female emulation of life-threatening habits long practiced by men, and the concomitant rise in their mortality rates, will eventually wipe out the seven or eight year longevity advantage they have long held over their male counterparts.

Six out of every 10 adult women in this country drink alcohol. Most are light to moderate drinkers, consuming anywhere from one drink a day to three drinks a week. Findings from research which focuses on the health consequences for these two groups are confusing and sometimes contradictory.[151] For example, it appears that *moderate* drinking for women reduces the risk of heart attack. In a study of more that 87,000 nurses ages 34 to 59, researchers reported that women who had one or two drinks a day had a 50 percent lower risk of heart attack, heart disease and the most common type of stroke than non-drinkers. Men enjoy similar heart-health benefits.[152] However, we have previously noted that some investigators have found a correlation between alcoholic consumption and breast cancer—even among women who drank only one or two alcoholic beverages per day. Moreover, according to the National Institute on Alcohol Abuse and Alcoholism more than one-fourth of alcohol abusers in the United States were women, mostly between the ages of 35 and 59. This third group is particularly at risk, exhibiting death rates significantly higher than its male counterparts.

A Word to the Wise Is Not Necessarily Sufficient

It is generally assumed that given proper information and education people will change their lifestyles to improve their health as well as their survival chances. It is a questionable assumption insofar as risk-taking is concerned. Since 1989, federal law has required that a warning label be placed on all alcoholic beverage containers, cautioning consumers about such risks as pregnancy complications and drunken driving. Public awareness of these cautionary labels is steadily increasing. There is little direct evidence to date, however, that such warnings are being heeded or are influencing behavior.[153] Perhaps in time, as public awareness continues to grow, more people will adopt the life-saving strategy of not mixing drinking with driving. Only time will tell.[154]

5

Stress and Its Associated Risks

Modern health research has moved away from a narrow physiological/biological/ chemical model for explaining human vulnerability to disease. This becomes rather apparent when we examine the relationship between stress, illness and survival. The relevant research literature is abundant, although by no means unanimous, in its understanding of the pathological, and sometimes beneficial, aspects of stress. Nor is there agreement about the differences among stress, tension, and strain. Hans Selye, the acknowledged pioneer of stress research, preferred to define it simply as the rate of wear and tear in the body. Here we focus on **stressors** that threaten our health and well-being, and that have the potential for curtailing our life chances. Stressors have been defined as "demands that tax or exceed the resources of the system or, to put it in a slightly different way, demands to which there are not readily available or automatic adaptive responses."[155]

The Fight or Flight Response. Stressful encounters trigger our physiological and psychological defenses which in turn prepare us for one of two classic, life-saving reactions—the so-called *fight or flight response*. These emanate from what is technically known as the sympathetic branch of our autonomic nervous system—which regulates much of the body's automatic reactions. When the resources of the system are overtaxed as, for example in the case of recurrent stressful episodes, or when neither the fight nor flight mechanisms are readily available, trouble can ensue. Urban dwellers of our large cities are often victims of such circumstances. Rudolph, for instance, describes the lot of New York City residents who daily and nightly feel pressured by local stresses which they feel helpless to alleviate or escape from. Consequently, their "...alarm reaction and the complex physiological changes it entails have nowhere to go but inward."[156] To avoid such deleterious effects, many residents have learned to launch each day prepared with alternative plans to resolve situations that might unavoidably confront them. Rudolph calls this *alternative power*. Many even take pride in their ability to "stay cool" under pressure and being able to overcome such challenges.

The beneficial effects of these alternatives and strategies take on added significance with the realization that stress not only can cause disease, but that it can also alter it. Studies done on both humans and animals indicate that prolonged, undue, or unrelieved strain and tension (anxiety?) are capable of triggering a variety of biochemical changes in our bodies, which in turn can affect our ability to remain healthy. The brain's hypothalamus is affected by stress and regulates the biochemical response of the body to its presence. This response can be lethal. Wilding, for example, reports that those who worked at the Kennedy Space Center during the pioneer days of the 1960's subsequently experienced a 50 percent higher incidence of sudden death and cardiovascular disorders than the general population.[157] We now know that how one copes with stress can affect the central nervous system, the cardiovascular system, and the immune system.

Stress And The Immune System. The effects on the immunity system can also be profound. It has been discovered, for example, that the way a heavy smoker reacts to the pressures of life affects the risk of developing lung cancer. In a recent study, it was noted that heavy smokers who coped well with stress did not develop lung cancer; those who did not cope well with the same types of stress did.[158] Similarly, speculation has emerged that those who carry the AIDS virus may help to trigger its active destruction by not coping well with stress. If this is substantiated, it may help provide a vital linkage between stress and the deterioration of the immunity system.

The Danger of Keeping A Stiff Upper Lip

At one point in his life Kenneth Lamott, a middle-aged man took the well-known Social Readjustment Rating Scale, which is designed to measure stress.[159] The many changes Lamott wasexperiencing in his life—going through a divorce, recovering from a cancer operation, losing a close friend who had died, moving to a new residence, and altering his basic lifestyle—gave him a high score on the scale. This placed him in a "trouble zone" and predicted that he had a 80 percent chance of becoming seriously ill, perhaps with a killing or crippling disease, within the next two years.[160]

Ironically, at the time Lamott was working against a deadline to complete a book entitled *Escape from Stress: How to Stop Killing Yourself.* By his own admission his life was ruled by deadlines, and he prided himself on never having missed one, no matter what it took out of him. Moreover, his personality was such that he tended to approach life with a "stiff upper lip," or, as he put it:

> I am a holder-in of emotion rather than a hanger-out—which is to say that my upbringing coupled with my peculiar mixture of genes and chromosomes conspire to keep personal feelings bottled up. One does not, I was taught, inflict one's private problems on other people. My upper lip remains stiff under the most extraordinary circumstances (p.30).

Hence, his outward reaction to critical events was generally one of tight-lipped or passive acceptance, and a tendency to expect the worse from the critical circumstances that impinged on his life.

Lamott decided that in order to avoid the dire results predicted by his scale score, he would have to change his approach to living. He resolved to do everything he could to survive, drawing on the knowledge he had gained while doing the research for his book. He knew that many scientists were convinced that the connection between stress and poor health had to do with our fight-or-flight reaction to various circumstances, in which adrenaline is quickly released into our bodies. When it and other hormones are continually pumped into our system in response to a variety of stress inducing stimuli, they eventually weaken our resistance to illness and disease. To counter this process, Lamott determined to exercise greater control of his circumstances. He moved to alter those aspects of his lifestyle, especially the tendency to be driven by deadlines, which could set off the fight-or-flight reaction. He knew from reading the relevant literature that work related stress, *per se*, was not what wore people down but rather, the stress of failure and frustration. He also learned that people who enjoy their work tend to be less vulnerable to serious disease than those who don't. Hence, when possible, he avoided undertakings in his work that he suspected would lead to dissatisfaction. He purposely slowed the hurried pace of his existence by building in periods of relaxation and practicing transcendental meditation. Though there were periodic relapses to the old destructive behavior patterns, over time he managed better to cope with stress and thereby achieve a healthier command over his life. It wasn't easy. It took practice and consistency. But it worked.

The Type "C" Personality

Certain elements of Lamott's personality—the stiff upper lip and pent-up feelings components—are also evident in what some have termed the Type C personality, one that is particularly prone to cancer.[161] It's also known as the "nice guy" personality, characterized by:

> the sort of person who wants to please others, even to the detriment of his own desires; the type who holds in his needs, frustrations and anger, and goes out of his way to avoid troubling friends, family or strangers. Some experts feel that such "niceness" is a coverup for a lack of self-esteem…The nice people are rather depressed. They seem to have lost hope of ever achieving what they want in life(p. 108).

Unlike the Type A personality discussed in an earlier chapter, the Type C personality exhibits a generally low level of emotional expressiveness. The reader may recall that the traits associated with the Type A individual included hostility, impatience, aggressiveness, and competitiveness. The Type C individual, in contrast, loathes expressing disruptive or hostile emotions, is afraid to be assertive, and prefers to be nice and compliant. Hence, much of what he feels, especially in the way of anger and frustration, remains bottled up.

Studies of some cancer patients reveal that those who tend to suppress negative emotions fare less well than those who openly express themselves. The latter group was often found to experience less aggressive tumor growth and a stronger immunologic response to the cancer. This suggests that how people handle their feelings can influence their anti-cancer immune defenses. Those who vent their feelings may be contributing to their survival. "It is widely recognized that cancer patients with a "fighting spirit"—and those who complain and agonize in the hospital—recover more often and more swiftly than the "good" or "no trouble" patients" (p.109). Increasingly, the bitching and agonizing, the demands for attention, in short the aggressive expression on the part of patients are being recognized as healthy indicators of their struggle to stay in charge of their situations.

The sense that one has some control over one's body and can fight for one's own recovery has emerged as a basic tenet of recovery and survival. Observations of a group of women with breast cancer found they could be divided into two categories according to their reactions following the diagnosis. One group was characterized by hopelessness, denial, and stoic acceptance—a sense of resignation about their fate. The other group exhibited a strong fighting spirit—they expressed a conviction that they could affect the outcome of their illness and were determined to fight to stay alive. When the two groups were followed up a decade later, the "fighters" clearly had the higher survival rate. The implication here is that:

If people with cancer can summon up an aggressive response in defense of themselves, with faith in the possibility of change, they might awaken their own disease-fighting mechanism. Likewise, if healthy individuals learn to do the same, it's possible that their disease-battling mechanisms will work more effectively to protect them from illness (p.158).

The reader should not misinterpret this conclusion. The words "might" and "possible" are meant to indicate just that. All that is being suggested is that, given the choice between throwing in the towel and succumbing to a life-threatening illness, or adopting an offensive posture to confront it, the latter option *might* lead to a positive outcome.

There is evidence that certain personality traits established early in life eventually become associated with certain diseases. On the basis of various prospective studies, in which personality data was collected *before* the victims succumbed to an illness, it has been suggested that cancer, asthma, heart-attack, stomach-ulcer, rheumatoid-arthritis, even urinary tract infections are each linked to distinct life-history and character traits.[162] However, despite the evidence linking personality to disease, some crucial questions remain unanswered. Analysts:

> ...still have only a tenous idea of how thoughts and emotions occur in the brain and how the brain in turn signals the body to alchemize the thoughts and emotions into somatic disease. Then there's the question of how personality interacts with other disease-risk factors, say the Type A personality and dietary cholesterol...Another unanswered question is why people with similar personality traits don't always end up with the same disease (p.66).

There is a general consensus that one is not born with these character traits. A person doesn't emerge from the womb as a Type C personality, which is amenable to alteration. The result can be a stronger body defense system which may lower the risk of cancer. There is general agreement that "C" type individuals would benefit from engaging in a process of introspection which eventually leads to a rediscovery and strengthening of their self concept. This process of self-discovery aims to get them back in touch with their physical and emotional needs and, if successful, results in a restructuring of priorities and goals which enable them to satisfy those needs. It is also important that they learn to monitor acute stress as a means of disease prevention. This includes developing a greater awareness of the feelings that accompany strain and tension, then seeking appropriate ways to express them.

Personality Hardiness

Some people seem to exhibit a strong resilience to stress. Workers in some high pressure occupations, for example, seem less vulnerable to illness than others in less demanding occupations. How does one account for the difference? Stress resistant people exhibit a set of personality characteristics which leads them to appraise events or circumstances differently from other persons. These health-protecting characteristics have been subsumed under the general rubric of *psychological hardiness*, which is composed of three major components: (a) openness to change and seeing it as a *challenge* and not a threat; (b) a sense of *commitment* to and involvement in what one is doing; and (c) a sense of *control* over life events and circumstances.[163],[164]

This set of attitudes can profoundly affect our health. People who could be rated high on these three attributes can be under great pressure and yet suffer fewer psychological problems and less physical illness.[165] Those who typically perceive life's stressful moments as a challenge, for example, are more likely to be physically healthy than those who see them as a calamity. How people define and experience change is important. A man who was laid off from his job, for instance, could define the situation in terms of personal rejection and the end of his career, or he could view this change (challenge) as an opportunity to find a new position, one better suited to his interests and abilities. People high on challenge are not afraid to take chances but at the same time avoid extreme types of risk-taking. They differ from those personality types who exhibit the trait of *excessive fearlessness*, a dangerous characteristic which can lead to premature death when such people fail to recognize that intense stress could be a signal to be very cautious.[166]

A second component of psychological hardiness entails a certain sense of commitment, characterized by people actively engaged in life.[167] They are not passive types who sit back on the fringe of things. Individuals who rate high on commitment tend to be engrossed in their work and families, as well as in their interpersonal relationships. They purposely seek to deal with their surroundings in the belief that they can significantly influence what takes place there. A high sense of commitment is correlated with greater stress tolerance capabilities and a healthier physical life.

Perhaps the most important element of personality hardiness in terms of mitigating the effects of stress is control. Control entails measures a person takes to change, adapt, or minimize the effects of pressure build-up. Such adaptations are usually behaviorally expressed, although they often can entail psychological or emotional adjustments. As Selye reminds us: "The outcome of our interactions with the environment depends just as much upon our reactions to the stressor as upon the nature of the stressor itself."[168] A wide body of literature supports the contention that a sense of control is related to how well one copes with stress, and the extent to which a lack of control becomes a threat to health and life. For example, we now know from reports of freed hostages and prisoners of war that, although faced with incredible deprivation and threats to their lives, they *actively* sought to maintain their morale acting to retain some semblance of control over what happened to them. Military survivors of prisoner-of-war camps:

> ...report a continued determination to carry the war to the enemy by bollix-ing his camp, disobeying his rules, upsetting everything they can, pretending to be feeble-minded, never learning the language, never cooperating, resisting, trying to escape, always trying to escape. They also carry on physical exercise instead of sitting there and waiting. They organize games, keeping hope up by this means, and keep busy through organizations and administration.[169]

On the other hand, those prisoners who chose an apathetic stance, who resigned themselves to the situation, and elected to simply wait until the Red Cross came to let them out, frequently died.[170]

In examining the complex relationship between stressful life events and psychological well-being, social scientists find it useful to employ the concepts of *external locus of control orientations* and *internal locus of control orientations*. Persons with external locus of control orientations are more fatalistic in outlook; they tend to believe they are at the mercy of their social environment and hence there is little they can do to overcome stressful events. Given that orientation, they are less apt to utilize available resources to cope with the circumstances in which they find themselves. They are also less likely to try to avoid or prepare for future problems. Persons with internal locus of control orientations, in contrast, believe that they can master or alter the environment. Hence, they are more apt to assume an active problem-solving approach to living that leads to coping behaviors that alter, prepare for, or avoid stressful events as they occur.[171]

Not only do people with a strong sense of control over life events contend significantly better with stress,[172] but they are more likely to engage in health-promoting behaviors.[173] The evidence continues to mount that a sense of low control, often involving what some term a *learned sense of helplessness*, is itself related to negative consequences for personal well-being, and can even lead to death.[174,175] Seeman and Seeman[176], for example, found that this sense of help-lessness can be a determinant of disease. In analysis of data from a large and representative sample of residents from a metropolitan area, they found that a strong sense of control, what they call "internality," was associated with a variety of behaviors and attitudes that were health-maintaining, including: taking positive steps to preserve personal well-being (for example, exercise, moderate alcohol consumption); avoiding negative habits (such as smoking); being more optimistic about the early treatment of cancer; having higher ratings on one's self-reporting of general health; indicating a lower frequency of acute, and even chronic, illness; being better able to manage a response to illness (for instance, the length of time staying in bed); and exhibiting less dependence on physicians.

If control is such an important factor, what does one do about life-threatening situations that are seemingly out of control? If we are passengers on a jumbo jet, is there anything that can be done in case of a crash? The answer is "yes" for some situations. Obviously, a fatal plane crash that will kill all onboard is just that, fatal. There is nothing one can do to survive such events, except to assume a neurotic avoidance of air transportation. Yet, accident investigations, such as the one surrounding a plane fire in Cincinnati showed that several passengers could have been saved had they counted the number of rows of seats they were from the exits. That would have alleviated the effects of smoke that obscured their vision when they stood upright. The person in a hotel room passively increases the chance of death by not checking exit routes and calculating how to escape in case of a fire. One can make it a matter of unmitigated policy not to get into a boat without a life jacket or a car without "buckling up." In other words, there are procedures that one can routinely follow in anticipating an emergency. Yet millions choose to do nothing at all due to any number of reasons—fatalism, a subconscious death wish, ignorance, laziness, or denial of a threat—to name a few. Whatever the reason, the failure to employ anticipatory strategies is an indication that many people underestimate the control they could have exercised in saving their own lives.

Sudden Death Syndrome

The importance of control is nowhere more acutely felt than at moments of extreme emotional trauma. Studies suggest that illness is more apt to develop at those points where people are having difficulty coping with significant changes in their lives. This is especially likely to occur when they feel overwhelmed by their problems and are predisposed to give up. Such experiences can also lead to the *sudden death syndrome,* whereby people die within minutes or hours of a major event in their lives as the result of acute emotional agitation. Engel identified and analyzed a large number of deaths that appeared to be associated with such incidents, and concluded they were due to one of four causes: (a) the disruption of a close human relationship or the anniversary of the death of a loved one; (b) situations of personal danger with threat of injury or loss of life, including fights, quarrels, struggles, or attacks; (c) emotional stress resulting from loss of status, self-esteem, or valued possessions, as well as circumstances producing disappointment, humiliation, failure, or defeat; (d) moments of intense feelings of joy or triumph. He emphasized that sudden death can occur when people "...are confronted with events that are impossible to ignore, either because of their abrupt, unexpected, or dramatic quality, or because of their intensity, irreversibility, or persistence."[177]

Nearly half of the cases fell into the first category—mortality due to the loss or disruption of a close relationship. Almost 4 out of 10 in this category died within the first two weeks after the loss of a loved one or after loved ones were exposed to danger. Two cases illustrate this pattern. A father was watching his two-year-old child in a wading pool, but his attention wandered and he became distracted. The child fell into the pool and drowned, and the father died moments later. A second case concerns a middle-aged woman who witnessed a truck accident involving her husband. She ran to his aid, and then collapsed and died, even though her husband had not been seriously injured.

The second category, which included about 37 percent of the cases, points to the fact that the dramatic and intense nature of sudden emotional impact can result in death even when one is actually spared from life-threatening physical encounters. In the cases that fell into this category, men were victims three times as often as women. The example is given of two close male friends who had a violent argument. While they didn't actually hit each other during this incident, one of the men suddenly collapsed and died. The other, who apparently had a history of heart disease, became acutely short of breath and then died shortly afterward. A person may emerge from a major automobile accident unhurt only to drop dead later when the realization of the immensity of the incident overwhelms him with a fatal outcome. Sometimes the acute psychological stress carries over to related incidents. A 50 year-old man lived though a major earthquake, only to die at his desk a few months later during a minor tremor. In some instances the excitement of witnessing a highly emotional drama can have deadly consequences. A journalist expired while photographing the drama of a rescue attempt to save a boy from an ice flow near Niagara Falls.

Others may suddenly drop dead at times of intensely felt disappointment, failure, defeat, loss of status, of self-esteem, or of highly valued possessions, as well as at moments of deeply felt joy or triumph. All the deaths that fit this third category involved males. Illustrative here was a 59-year-old college president who was forced out of his position. He died at the ceremony installing his replacement.

The fourth category of people, those succumbing during moments of joy or triumph, although involving the smallest number of victims, is perhaps particularly puzzling. An example here is the middle-aged minister who was exhilarated about the opportunity to talk to the President of the United States over a radio call-in show. The minister had a fatal heart attack shortly after the conversation. In another case, an elderly man died of a coronary attack after winning the daily double.

One could easily conclude that *any* exceptionally emotionally charged situation carries with it the potential for unanticipated annihilation. However, a more rational conclusion, and the one that seems to derive not only from these cases but from the medical literature is as follows:

> For the most part, the victims are confronted with events that are impossible to ignore, either because of their abrupt, unexpected, or dramatic quality or because of their intensity, irreversibility, or persistence. The individual experiences or is threatened with overwhelming excitation. Implicit, also is the idea that he no longer has, or no longer believes that he has, mastery or control over the situation or himself, or fears that he may lose what control he has (p. 154).

The categories of sudden cardiac death just discussed underscore the significance of *control* as a component of survival. The opposite feelings of helplessness and hopelessness, or of just giving up in the face of traumatic circumstances or perceived impasses, can set the stage for an unanticipated and sudden demise. At times of trauma, we must call on one of our basic emergency systems: quick motor activity (fight or flight), or inactivity and disengagement (a more passive acceptance, or withdrawal). One must control the assessment of the trauma to determine which of the two systems to use. Since these systems are reciprocal, a person under severe distress must realize that the response chosen can contain elements of both emergency systems. The important matter is that people quickly appraise the situation, and then attempt to regulate his response. This, of course, is easier said than done, as the following example illustrates. A 60-year-old woman was working at a motel desk when a menacing-looking man suddenly burst in and demanded money. Terrified, she quickly obeyed. The robber fled and she called the police. Later, upon leaving for the police station, she began gasping for air and clutching her chest. She was hurriedly taken to the hospital.

Though she had no history of heart disease or hypertension, at the hospital she began to experience erratic hearth rhythms. She died two hours after the robbery. The robber was eventually caught. At the trial, expert testimony linking her fright to the subsequent heart damage convinced the jury to find the robber guilty of felony-murder. "The case is one of the few in which a defendant has been convicted of scaring someone to death."[178]

Why certain persons suffer fatal consequences from surges of cardiovascular activity brought on by highly emotional events, while others do not, is a difficult question to answer. It has been suggested by that people who over time experience repeated traumatic emotional reactions, may produce damage to the heart tissue which in turn predisposes them to sudden death. A similar suggestion has been made regarding individuals that have been exposed to very long periods of stress over many years. Such circumstances are thought to lead to a chronic elevated level of psychoendrocrine hormones in the body, which eventually affect their cardiovascular health. Others have proposed that the answer may lie in identifying certain chemicals in the brain which, in abnormal amounts, interfere with the brain's ability to regulate the accelerated heartbeat and associated blood pressure surges produced by emotional stress. At this point, those people most susceptible to the factors that trigger unusual *ventricular fillibration* may be able to avoid its lethal outcomes by taking blood-pressure or anti-arrhythmic medications, or through behavioral counseling and training in relaxation techniques designed to alter an extreme panic responses.

6

Strategies for Dealing with Stress

Peter G. Hanson, author of *The Joy of Stress*, exhorts the public not to hide from stresses; instead "go out and challenge new ones." While some may never be convinced of the positive effects of this approach, others could increase their survival chances by accepting the fact that life is inherently filled with daily risks or tensions. Thus, one should not waste time and energy in trying to avoid or escape from such pressures. Hans Selye put it most succinctly when he wrote: "Complete freedom from stress is death." He also observed that we tend to misuse the term stress in common parlance. "Any kind of normal activity—a game of chess or even a passionate embrace—can produce considerable stress without causing harmful effects." Hence, he preferred to denote damaging stress as *distress*.[179] One might distinguish between intermittent and persistent stress. It is the latter that is apt to lead to such negative consequences as heart disease, strokes, chronic indigestion, stomach ulcers and migraine headaches. Moreover, it generally will be the case that no single element of daily living will be solely responsible for all of one's anxiety and tension. Rather, a combination of factors will more likely tip the scale toward stress overload.

For some, daily tension goes with the job and is expected as, for example, in the case of air traffic controllers. Given the nature of their work, it should come as no surprise to learn that they develop hypertension much more frequently than people in other occupations. However, the risk of illness or disease from being in a high pressure occupation is not inevitable. Kobasa's study of lawyers, for example, did not find the expected relationship between stress and sickness.[180] Why? She speculated that lawyers are socialized to view pressure as intrinsic to their work and careers. Therefore, they might very well internalize the notion that their best work is actually produced under such conditions. Given these expectations, one may not find the same relationship between work-related tension and illness so often among attorneys as for some other occupational groups. Business executives, for example, are constantly reminded that stress will kill them. Hence, they develop the attitude that it can be detrimental to their work performance and health and, therefore, should be avoided or minimized via biofeedback techniques, exercise, or through other outlets.

Compartmentalization. Even when people live with a healthy expectation of stress, they must also learn to compartmentalize emotional tension especially that associated with their work. The old adage of "leaving one's job at the office" is proper advice for promoting longevity. Army officers, for example, are much more prone to mental and physical illness than business executives. Kobasa attributes the greater vulnerability of the officers, in part, to the total institutional character of army life, which embraces every aspect of their existence. Within that inclusive environment it is very difficult for them to isolate their military careers from the rest of their lives. Interestingly, these officers also scored lower on commitment than the attorneys or business executives.[181]

Social Support. Social support is related to the ability to cope with stress, but the strength of such support is closely linked to one's personality and commitment.[182] A detailed discussion of the importance of social networks to the maintenance of mental and physical health can be found in the following chapter. Here we simply note that strong, affirming social relationships, may enhance an individual's ability to improve well-being or to counter the potentially adverse effects of stressful life events.[183] Conversely, the absence of strong social ties can greatly amplify a person's vulnerability to the unhealthy effects of tension. Prolonged absence of social support or intimate relations with others apparently can exert a particularly detrimental effect on one's physical or mental health. As far back as the early 1940's, Cannon[184] noted that one of the major causes of death from the ancient voodoo practices was the complete isolation victims experienced after a "hex" was placed on them.

This relationship between stress and isolation has been studied in Israel. Pines[185] looked at the relative isolation of urban children at times of military bombings and compared them with children who experienced such bombings while living in a context of a kibbutz settlement. Children who lived in the kibbutz experienced less mental stress and anxiety during these attacks than their urban counterparts, who felt more isolated from others. When these events occurred, the kibbutz children were led to a shelter where they were assured of not having to be alone; "shelters that were familiar to them, where educational programs and life went on pretty much as usual." No such assurance was available to children who lived in the cities, who: "accustomed to living in family units, were suddenly taken to alien and somewhat disordered community shelters; their daily routine was upset."

Further understanding the connection between social networks, stress, and personality comes from research which focuses on the reasons people establish relationships. It appears that one's *motivation* for seeking social ties may be an important factor in relation to stress. McClelland[186] found that some people sought certain relations to satisfy a strong desire for power. Those who pursued social ties for this reason *and* were greatly inhibited about expressing this need for power were the most vulnerable to illness. At times of stress, such people feel an inner restraint that frustrates their ability to act. As he put it: "The equivalent at the personality level would appear to be a strong disposition to act assertively which is simultaneously checked by an inner desire for control and restraint."[187] Thus, in a study by him and an associate, it was found that college students who sought social ties for affiliation purposes did not experience the same degree of severe illness under stress as their counterparts who were motivated by a need for power, but were also inhibited in expressing this need. Indeed, those students who exhibited a high need for power and were able to express that motivation openly were relatively protected against "power\achievement stress." They may be somewhat similar to the outspoken business man who stated: "I don't *get* ulcers, I *give* them."[188]

The Work Environment

Another factor that affects the relationship between stress and illness is the work environment. Not surprisingly, it's been found that "…people who have little control over their jobs, such as cooks, garment stitchers and assembly-line workers, have higher rates of heart disease than people who can dictate the pace and style of their work."[189] Jobs which involve high psychological strain but low job control (little decision-making power), carry with them the potential for greater health risks. People in certain service occupations which do not allow them to exercise much choice over how they relate to the client are high in stress—for example, telephone operators or nurse's aides. In many of these jobs the workers are embedded within a large organization with rules that restrain them from responding to client needs in the way they would like. This can be frustrating. In contrast, people who possess decision-making power over the work process—scientists or skilled machinists, for instance—tend to exhibit comparatively low stress levels. Because they are more apt to feel confident that they have a strategy for mastering work-related problems, and because they are in charge of deciding when to apply such strategies, they are more likely to have a reduced-stress response.[190] The demand\control context of one' occupation appears to be so paramount that its negative effects on health are similar to those of smoking or an elevated serum cholesterol level.

Significant Life Events

Significant life events can also play a role in increasing the effect of stress, thereby leading to possible changes in health. For various reasons not all major life events or transitions affect everyone in the same manner. That is, major life events and role transitions have been shown to produce a wide range of effects on the mental and physical health of individuals. Wheaton has noted that the search for the causes of this differential impact of life events has produced two major research models or traditions.[191] The first relies on what she calls the *differential vulnerability* argument, "in which differences in coping resources or strategies, ongoing dispositional qualities, or social locations determine the impact of events." This approach has also generated a related tradition which emphasizes the buffering effects of social support. A second tradition is based on the contention "that events vary in stressfulness because of differences in such characteristics as undesirability, uncontrollability, unpredictability, and event magnitude." This has been labelled the *trait approach* because it suggests that one can identify the most significant life events affecting a person through an array of event characteristics that specify stress potential. The widely used Holmes—Rahe scale would be illustrative here. Wheaton rejects the presumption that life transitions are inherently or universally stressful. She argues that prior role circumstances largely determined the impact of subsequent events. Hence, she adopts a third so-called *contextual approach* in order to understand the variations in people's responses to similar life transitions. It emphasizes the importance of prior chronic role stress in determining those responses.[192]

> Chronic role stress is likely to be a central feature in understanding individual differences in the experience of a life transition. The meaning of a divorce after a "bad" marriage will surely be quite different than a divorce after a "good" marriage. Getting fired from a job where you hate the boss or that is excessively dangerous will lead to different mental health consequences than getting fired from a secure, interesting job with ample opportunities for promotion. When a long-term alcoholic dies, his or her spouse is likely to feel some relief from the burden of a difficult caretaker role (p.210).

This suggests that the potentially harmful effects of major transitions can be mitigated by the presence of previous difficulties.

This has been characterized as a *stressful event as stress relief* model. Using data from a national survey of Canadian adults, Wheaton analyzed the impact of a number of life and role transitions over time—job loss, divorce, premarital break-up, retirement, widowhood, children moving out of the house, first marriage, job promotion, and having a child—and found considerable support for this contextual argument. He concludes that "the stress potential of an event is neither an inherent characteristics of the event nor a result of "coping" strategies, but instead is a product of the social environment prior to the occurrence of the transition." (p. 220). Hence, in some instances, perhaps many, a transition circumstance may present an opportunity for the person to remove themselves from a tense situation into a more manageable and even more positive environment.

Life Crisis Events. Analysts have focused on the extent to which Life Crisis Events (LCEs) impact on our psychological and physical well-being. LCEs have been defined as "...objective occurrences of sufficient magnitude to bring about change in the usual activities of those who experience them."[193] Although investigators distinguish among a wide range of such occurrences, perhaps the most crucial are loss of spouse or family member, divorce or separation, loss of job, retirement, change in social status, major financial difficulty, and, of course, change in one's own health or that of a loved one.

For our purposes, we need emphasize only three ideas: First, both negative, for instance, loss of a job, and positive, for example, a promotion at work, life events have the potential for generating stress. Second, how one perceives and copes with life events influences the possible deterioration in life chances—by adverse psychological and/or physical consequences. Such outcomes can range from suicide to a propensity to be involved in auto accidents to a more subtle, yet direct, impact on well-being, including depression, alcoholism, and cardiovascular problems.[194] Third, as with any tension, the effect of LCEs is contingent on one's prior circumstances and past experience of dealing with stress, as well as how one utilizes available resources to deal with present conditions. In the long run, one's health and survival may not be so much affected by life events, *per se*, but rather by how well one has learned to respond to them in an appropriate fashion.

Additional Stress Reduction Strategies

We have underscored the linkage between stress and its resulting harm on health, as well as the psychosocial factors that affect this linkage. Awareness of these factors can be instrumental in minimizing if not avoiding negative repercussions, provided the individual acts on this awareness. Moreover, there are specific behaviors and strategies that one can utilize to "short-circuit" the link between stress and disease, including the following[195].

(a) *Time and the development of priorities.* Organization of time is an excellent technique for controlling stress. Implicit here is the notion of time as a valued personal possession. "Does thou love life?" wrote Benjamin Franklin. "Then do not squander time, for that is the stuff life is made of." Although most of us recognize that we have a finite allotment of time on this planet, we nevertheless thoughtlessly squander away good amounts of it. We fail to appreciate that well-organized time allows us to get our work done with less wear and tear on our emotions and less strain on our health. The underlying purpose of good time management is to increase our "disposable" time so that there is a healthy balance between work related activities and those directed towards other life goals. One way to achieve that balance is to establish priorities with respect to tasks and objectives. By doing so people are in a better position to avoid anxiety over getting things done that, sometimes upon closer investigation, are really not that important or can be delegated to others.

A clear sense of priorities enables a person to view pressure in a more rational perspective. Unnecessary concern over matters of little consequence is wasted emotional energy. Tension from high priority matters can be effectively dealt with by focusing behavior to systematically work through these situations. "The paradox of time management, as of other aspects of life, is that greater control means greater freedom to do the things we want to do. By making the most of time, we can go a long way towards making the most of our lives."[196]

(2) *Stress avoidance.* One way to prevent stress from being pathological is to avoid it. Avoidance does not mean assuming a posture of "staying in a rut" to evade challenge. It does not mean, for example, becoming a "couch potato" mesmerized by indiscriminate television-viewing. In fact, such passive escapism can produce negative consequences, for instance, boredom and loneliness. Rather, avoidance here means utilizing positive strategies to circumvent situations or conditions that are stress provoking. Examine daily situations that are tension-producing and actively seek to avoid them if possible, or modify the circumstances to lessen the impact of stress. Leave home for work ten minutes earlier to avoid heavy traffic. Bring a brown bag to work to avoid having to go to lunch with an irritating co-worker. The key is to avoid stress where possible and to learn to invoke positive behaviors where it cannot be avoided.

(c) *Get Away.* It is important to have a set time to relax and get one's mind off of stressful situations. On a daily basis, this can be going for a walk, unplugging the phone and television for quiet time alone or with the family. Contemporary environments daily bombard us with irritating decibels of noise which, if continued at certain intensities, provoke unhealthy physiological reactions—rises in blood pressure, increased heartbeats, rushes of adrenalin, and so on. Periodic periods of silence can be therapeutic. A quiet walk in the park or woods, or a stroll along a lake or ocean shore, can have a calming and rehabilitative effect.

People are often surprised to discover that moments of solitude can have recuperative consequences, allowing us to momentarily escape the pettiness in life and instead focus on our inner identity. Solitude can set the stage for "interior dialogues" between our warring "congregation of selves," and eventually result in a greater understanding of our feelings, perceptions, and behavior. It may, if consciously utilized to achieve growth and greater maturity, even rejuvenate the human spirit for survival.[197]

On a long term basis, getting out of town is sometimes essential to coping with strains of our daily existence. Vacations must be a priority, but they need not be three-week-long treks across country. In fact, some experts believe that frequent short holidays might be better than one long vacation. Getting away for the weekend several times a year—experiencing a change of scenery—can be extremely beneficial.

Implicit here is the management of time. Those personalities who find it difficult if not impossible to separate work time from rest and recreation time often court mental and physical fatigue. These "workaholics" fail to appreciate the restorative benefits of doing something different from their every-day work during their off-hours. Never being able to "let the job go" for very long, never giving leisure the high priority it deserves, can in the long run be detrimental to one's health and well-being. Especially during the later stages of the life-cycle, middle-age and beyond, a diversified "leisure portfolio" that embraces "some exercise or sports, some creative craft or hobby (or both), some entertainment, some socializing, some travel, and study in some field unrelated to your work," becomes an essential strategy for sustaining a quality existence. Without such a strategy, the well known debilitative consequences of boredom are apt to set in. Boredom, it has been said, "creates more drunkards than thirst, more gamblers than greed, and more suicides than despair."[198]

As is the case with so many aspects of the human condition, the use or abuse of leisure time, whether it is a blessing or a curse, ultimately becomes a matter of personal choice. Used wisely, it can move us closer to the achievement of our human potential and to savoring life to its fullest. In other words, our attitudes and activities surrounding leisure time can help sustain the belief that life is indeed worth living.

(d) *Exercise.* As we noted in an earlier chapter, one of the most immediate things people can do to lessen the impact of stress is physical activity. It not only helps to get one's mind off stress, but it also has a direct physiological consequence which mitigates the effect of stress. Physical exercise helps the release of endorphins which are, quite literally, the body's opiates that help to reduce depression resulting from stress. Parenthetically, most physical exercise helps to enhance one's self-image by improving physical appearance and body tone. A positive self-image in turn helps to increase one's level of confidence and control in handling a variety of tense situations.

(e) *Expand interpersonal networks.* Developing friendships and maintaining close primary ties can be a very important influence on the length and quality of life. This is especially true for coping with stress. Loners are more likely to suffer mental disorders than more socially active people, and are more likely to die prematurely. By expanding one's interpersonal networks, one can enjoy the pleasant and therapeutic company of friends who can offer emotional support as well as helpful advice. Breaking a sense of isolation by talking out problems with friends, sometimes even acquaintances, can be very effective in contending with stress.

(f) *Proper diet.* When a people are at their proper weight, they usually has a better feeling about how they look, thereby reducing a major source of anxiety—that of being under-or-overweight. However, a proper diet of balanced meals, fiber, protein, and low cholesterol also increases the positive effect that nutrition can have on the body chemistry. This chemistry must be especially maintained under times of stress, when one's immune system is more susceptible to disease.

(g) *Use of relaxation techniques.* There are a variety of behaviors that can be done throughout the day to reduce the physiological ramifications of prolonged or intense anxiety. These can often be done in one's home or office. By slowly deep-breathing and exhaling for five minutes, one can retard the anxiety-provoked breathing rhythm produced by stress. By tightening one's muscles, then slowly relaxing them, tension can also be reduced. For many people, twenty minutes of meditation a day can produce a similar effect.

(h) *Biofeedback and hypnosis.* Biofeedback, through the use of electronic skin sensors, can assess the extent of stress as it increases physical tension. Therapists can then advise a person on certain techniques, for example, imagining a pleasant setting, that help alleviate the problem. Also, hypnosis can be very effective in coping with stress, and many people can be taught the techniques of self-hypnosis.

We know that two people can react to the same situation in quite different ways, depending on their own temperament and past training and experience. A given situation can be viewed as threatening by one and not the other. Construction workers on high-rise buildings or very tall bridges respond differently to those environments than persons afraid of heights. For some people, life is filled with annoying and anxiety provoking hassles, especially on the job, whose *cumulative* effect can be more damaging than a major life event. For others, the relentless pressure of life in a poverty-stricken ghetto are apt to be more related to high health risks than frictions on the job.[199] For one spouse, divorce and its aftermath can mean hopelessness and despair, while for the other it can signal freedom, opportunity and renewed feelings of happiness. Developing a conscious awareness of those conditions which might trigger a stress response, along with the ability to employ some basic coping skills, can go a long way toward neutralizing potential debilitating effects. In the final analysis, it may be that "far more important than the trials and tribulations in one's life is how one deals with them" (p.50).

The Two-Edged Sword of Emotions: Anger

Our lives are filled with emotionally provoking encounters. Whether such encounters can damage our health and threaten our survival greatly depends on how we manage the encounter and the emotion. At one time, conventional wisdom had it that the spontaneous ventilation of feelings effected a positive contribution to our mental and physical well-being. Conversely, it was argued that people who totally repressed such aggressive feelings would eventually become victims of hypertension. Most emotions, it turns out, have this quality of a two-edged sword. Medical researchers, for example, have accumulated strong evidence that *frequent, intense, and prolonged* anger can have adverse health consequences. In an previous chapter we noted studies of the Type A personality which found that those males with a high level of anger (underlying this anger were attitudes of deep hostility and distrust of others) experienced more severe arteriosclerosis and a much greater death rate than men with a lower levels of anger. The problem is, such consequences can result from either the expression *or* the repression of anger. Too much of one mode of response or the other can be equally unhealthy—both are capable of releasing damaging amounts of adrenaline into our bloodstream.

Resolution of this dilemma—to vent anger or suppress it—lies in striving for a balanced, controlled response, one that avoids the pattern of continuous, excessive anger. Some people are able to successfully employ the technique of *cognitive therapy*, which entails rethinking our angry responses and then deliberately restructuring our attitudes and perceptions of situations which trigger that response. This involves a strategy of exercising conscious control over your initial reactions, taking a moment to review them in a rational fashion, and then channeling them into constructive actions.[200] Taking constructive action to resolve one's anger or to avoid its escalation can have positive consequences for our health. However, it is not easy to curb rage or to alter habitual responses to irritating encounters. People who have developed a chronic pattern of anger find it especially difficult, and may have to resort to *drug therapy* as a preventive measure to block the impact of "anger hormones" on their coronary systems. Letting anger get the best of us can lead to unwelcome outcomes. As one researcher put is:

> The Bible, from the Old Testament to the New Testament, is filled with all these injunctions: to love rather than hate people, to not let the sun set on your anger. I'm not saying that you shouldn't get angry just because the bible says you shouldn't, because you should realize that if you let your anger get the better of you, it's going to be bad for you. It's going, perhaps to make you sick. Maybe it will kill you.[201]

Summary

The evidence that stress affects both the quality and length of life is constantly accumulating and, in fact, is overwhelming. In this chapter several common strategies have been suggested that have proven to be effective in coping with this problem—at least for some people. Although anxieties and tensions are a part of everyday living, a person can exert some control to minimize if not prevent them from influencing the etiology of disease and other pathologies. It is very difficulty to permanently alter one's underlying personality structure. It is much easier to learn and adapt certain behavioral techniques—those associated with psychological hardiness, for example—which would protect us from stress-induced disabilities and which allow us to become increasingly stress-resistant.[202] Given the pressures of daily living, the implementation of routine coping strategies appears essential to a continued healthy existence.

7

Social Networks: One Key to Life Preservation

There is substantial evidence that people who are embedded in networks of social relationships exhibit the lowest mortality risk. Consensus is building in the scientific community that these connections play a critical role in the determination of health status. For example, research findings suggest the harmful health consequences associated with stressful life events can be reduced through support from social networks. In addition there are strong indications that social and community ties may play a role in the etiology of disease. One team of researchers[203] looked at the impact of a range of social ties and networks in relation to mortality from all causes in a large sample of people who were followed over a nine-year period. It was found that those who lacked such ties were more likely to die in the follow-up period than those with more extensive contacts. This association was independent of self-reported physical health status at the time of the initial survey, year of death, socioeconomic status, and health practices, such as smoking, utilization of preventive health services, as well as a cumulative index of health practices.

In examining the effects on mortality of increasing social isolation, the investigators constructed a Social Network Index, which took into account not only the size of a person's network, but also their relative importance. Analyses of the age-and-sex specific mortality rates from all causes revealed "a consistent pattern of increased mortality rates associated with each decrease in social connection" (p. 190). Even more significant is their finding that this relationship exists independently of several variables traditionally expected to be predictors of mortality. That is, they found this pattern to hold true independent of one's health status, social class, smoking status, obesity, alcoholic beverage consumption, and physical activity. This provides strong support for the argument that social and community ties significantly affect a person's life-expectancy potential; "that social factors may influence host resistance and affect vulnerability to disease in general" (p. 203).

While the above study is exceptionally revealing, it also leaves many questions unanswered. One such question is whether there is some minimal number of possible relationships that an individual must have in order to avoid falling into a particular risk category. They found, for example, that unmarried respondents with many friends and relatives had mortality rates equal to married subjects with fewer contacts with friends and relatives. Indeed, it did not seem to matter whether the contacts were among friends or among relatives. It was only when either of these sources of contacts was absent that a significant increase took pace in the risk of death during the follow-up period. In other words: "It was only in the presence of mounting social disconnection, when individuals failed to have links in several different spheres of interaction, that mortality rates rose sharply" (p. 201).

The mechanisms by which *social network embeddedness* influences health status and subsequent death have yet to be specified. The leaders of the above study found that social isolation was associated with overall mortality as well as specific causes of ischemic heart disease, cancer, cerebrovascular and circulatory diseases, diseases of the digestive and respiratory system, accidents, and suicides. They reason that there are probably several *pathways* that could lead from social isolation to illness:

> ...One pathway might be through the use of health practices which may lead to poor health consequences...A second pathway may be through psychological responses to isolation such as depression or changed coping and appraisal processes...Another pathway might lead directly from social isolation to physiological changes in the body which increase general susceptibility to disease (p. 202).

While any one of these pathways, or some combination of them, could lead to increased morbidity, the specific mechanisms by which they are capable of doing so, by which they are translated into such outcomes, remains far from clear. What is clear is that social circumstances, such as social isolation, can have pervasive health consequences and affect our vulnerability to disease.

The Broken Heart Syndrome

Although the actual dynamics of mediating factors between social events and disease are not known, perhaps no event has been more studied than the loss of a family member. Analysts in the United States and abroad have found that a death in the family increases the probability of premature demise among the remaining members. Typically, these studies match and compare families who have suffered a bereavement during the past year with families who have not. The results generally reveal a death rate among surviving family members significantly greater than that observed among families who had not encountered a loss. Moreover, one of these investigations found that death rate increased among those relatives closest to the deceased, that is, among remaining spouses and children.[204] It also revealed that the subsequent risk was significantly higher for males that for females, and that if the death was sudden, accidental, or unanticipated, the death rate among the survivors doubled.

One explanation offered to account for these findings involves the notion of a **broken heart syndrome**, suggesting that loneliness and grief can so overwhelm certain individuals as to affect fatally their hearts.[205] Durkheim[206] is perhaps the best known early sociologist to emphasize the relation between widowhood and a particular type of death-related grief and the impact of widowhood on direct self-destruction. In his view, suicide following the loss of a mate reflects the consequences of what he termed *domestic anomy*: "A family catastrophe occurs which affects the survivor. He is not adapted to the new situation in which he finds himself and accordingly offers less resistance to suicide" (p. 259). Indeed, there is considerable data showing that suicide rates are higher among the widowed in comparison to the married. The evidence also suggests that the trauma of widowhood might weaken the resistance to other causes of death besides suicide.

The idea that severe grief can somehow damage the heart is actually an old one that can be dated to antiquity. It gained some scientific credence from observations that survivors, usually a spouse, sometimes die rather unexpectedly following the death of a marital partner. Autopsy reports would then reveal that the survivor had succumbed to some form of heart disease. Sometimes, the death of a spouse aggravates an already present heart condition in the survivor, leading to fatal results. Such instances add empirical support to our intuitive perception that the emotional and psychological consequences of loss and severe grief can affect both our ability and our will to live. Indeed, there is evidence of a psychological state termed the *giving-up-complex*.[207] A person reaching this psychological state feels that he is no longer able to cope with a situation, and then develops strong feelings of helplessness and hopelessness. At this point, he becomes unusually vulnerable to the onset of disease and even death. For example, if he is predisposed to diabetes, then the disease may appear during this moment of stress.[208]

An example of this phenomenon of the broken heart is the case of the former prime minister of Israel, Manachem Begin. His wife of 43 years die and, from that point on, there was a visible decline in his health and spirits, and he became something of a recluse, all of which was widely commented upon in the mass media. Mental health professionals, of course, know that it is not uncommon for a powerful man such as Begin to become despondent at the loss of a wife on whom he depended for emotional support for such a long time. The Executive Director of the Bereavement and Loss Center of New York notes that such reactions are often seen in high-ranking executives who lose their wives after a long marriage. Deprived of the one person to whom they could freely reveal their physical or emotional frailties, they soon experience "the loneliness of command, the increasing isolation, the ill health, self doubt.[209] Begin, by the way, also falls in this special high-risk group of survivors because he was 70 years old at the time and suffered from cardiac and circulatory problems. Moreover, men in similar situations are often reluctant to admit the need for or to seek professional help. They represent a generation of husbands heavily dependent on their spouses for physical, emotional, and other kinds of support. When that primary support is removed through death, they almost literally become heartbroken, and often die prematurely.[210]

The broken heart syndrome, while being increasingly recognized among the lay and scientific community alike, does not yield to a simple pattern of etiology. Up to the current decade, most researchers were in agreement with Parkes'[211] critical assessment:

> The fact that bereavement may be followed by death from heart disease does not prove that grief is itself a cause of death. We do not even know whether bereavement causes the illness or simply aggravates a condition that would have occurred anyway. Perhaps bereaved people tend to smoke more or to alter their diet in a way that increases their liability to coronary thrombosis. Even if emotional factors are directly implicated, we still have to explain how they affect the heart. Stress is known to produce changes in the blood pressure and heart rate, in the flow of blood through the coronary arteries and in the chemical constituents of the blood. Any of these changes could play a part in precipitating clotting within a diseased coronary artery and thereby produce a coronary thrombosis, but without further research, we can only speculate.

Recent evidence suggests that people who die from a "broken heart" may have experienced a reduction in their body defenses against disease that was brought on by grief. In a study of men whose wives had died of breast cancer, it was found that they experienced a significant decline in the activity of *lymphocytes*, which are white blood cells involved in the body's disease-fighting system.[212] This decline in lymphocyte activity occurred shortly after the wife's demise and failed to return to its former level even after a year had passed. Interestingly, while other studies have shown that bereaved persons feel sicker, spend more time in hospitals, and use alcohol, cigarettes, and tranquilizers more than persons who are not bereaved, such was not the case here. Rather, the subjects "did not report major or persistent changes in diet or activity levels or in the use of medications, alcohol, tobacco, or other drugs, and no significant changes in weight were noted" (p.337).

Diminished lymphocyte activity, then, may be an important element in the biosocial chain of reactions to the bereavement process which influences the health of survivors.[213] This finding adds to the accumulating evidence that immunity may be altered as a consequence of the bereavement experience and thereby contribute to subsequent morbidity and morality. While it has not been established that bereavement can directly cause disease, the available data suggests that loss reactions do contribute to the epidemiology of stress-related diseases. There is little question that, under certain circumstances, pathological patterns of grieving can develop and have devastating negative effects on the survivor's physical and emotional health.[214] The processes by which this occurs are not yet well understood, but the idea that grief and a broken heart can cause premature death is gaining acceptance among the lay and scientific communities.[215]

A number of alternative hypotheses or explanations has been offered to account for the increased mortality risk of surviving spouses, including: (a) *Homogamy.* The idea here is that "there is a tendency for the fit to marry the fit, and the unfit the unfit," with the latter situation producing some kind of marital disease association; (b) *Common infection.* Here, the suggestion is that both the husband and the wife may succumb to the same infectious disease. This notion of mutual infection may have some validity, for example, in the case of tuberculosis, influenza, or pneumonia; (c) *Joint unfavorable environment.* The proposal here is that the unfavorable environment which led to the demise of one spouse may significantly influence the death of the other; (d) *Loss of care.* The implication here is that, for a variety of reasons, survivorship adaptation may be more difficult for the husband, especially the older husband. Its been suggested that the widower's ability to resist disease is impaired by the loss of care and attention formerly provided by his wife. British scientists some years ago spoke of the widower becoming "malnourished" following the demise of his spouse.[216] Even earlier American researchers focusing on our older population offered a similar explanation, noting that:

> A life time of close association with a woman whose complementary activities form the basis of a home now requires the most basic revision for which the widower may be wholly unprepared…The vinculum that is marriage is disengaged by death and the widower may find himself incapable of remaking his life into an integrated whole.[217]

The argument here is that the older widower becomes vulnerable to demoralization and incapacitation in the absence of the socio-emotional support provided by the former spouse: (e) *The desolation effect.* In a related fashion, some make a distinction between isolation and desolation, with the latter viewed as having the more deleterious consequences for the survivor.[218] In general, isolation refers to the state of being separated from others, of being alone. Desolation, on the other hand, refers to feelings of abandonment and loneliness. Survivorship adaptation, it is argued, is impeded by intense or prolonged states of desolation. These conditions of unaltered sadness and melancholy presumably have the consequence of diminishing the normal probabilities for survival. One strongly suspects that it is for this reason that most societies have instituted rules and rituals designed, at least in part, to reintegrate bereaved individuals and to assist them in making a satisfactory adjustment to their new status.

The above suggests that grief can carry with it the potential for early demise. However, the loss of a spouse is apparently more devastating to men than it is to women. That is to say, men whose wives have died are much more likely to die earlier than men of the same age who are still married. A major long-term project confirms that the death of a husband, on the other hand, has little or no effect on the mortality rate of wives.[219] It also uncovered a link between marriage and longevity by finding that remarriage increased a male's chances of living longer. The study involved a 12-year survey of widowed people. For both sexes, the impact of spousal loss was slight during the first year. However, in the ensuing years, widowed men had a 28 percent greater mortality rate than their married male counterparts; between ages 55 and 65, their mortality rate was 60 percent higher.[220]

How does one account for the lower survival capability among widowers? Why are women less affected by the loss of a husband than vice-versa? The researchers speculate that the absence of the marital partner affects a man's quality of life in many more ways than in the case of a widow. They seem to be invoking the *loss of care hypothesis* in stating that "even if he joins a club or some other social activity, something is always going to be missing—someone to pay attention to him, to go out with him."[221] The effect of the wife's death on the husband appears to reflect a chronic, long-term problem of being alone, rather than an immediate response to the death itself. Women, on the other hand, may simply have greater capacities for adapting to change. In other words, it may be "that the same physiological and psychological differences that give females greater longevity than males also act to make females more resistant to the stress of widowhood."[222] In addition, women are more likely than men to socialize other women into the widowed role and into widowhood networks, and to develop new friendships, all of which have positive consequences [223]

Social factors, then, appear to play a significant role in the higher death risk of males and may help explain their greater vulnerability to the stresses of widowhood, especially among older groups. For example, in one study that compared the critical problems confronting an aged, married, and widowed group, the widowers emerged as the most socially isolated subjects.[224] This was especially true among those who were older, relatively uneducated, and residing in a rural environment. Another factor that led to social isolation was poor health, which sometimes caused a widower to be confined to his home and consequently limited his social contacts. In addition, in comparison to other marital statuses, widowers were *least* likely to be living with children, to have a high degree of kin interaction or to be satisfied with extended family relationships. They also were *least* likely to receive from or give to children various forms of assistance, or to have friends either in or outside the community, or to be satisfied with their opportunities to be with close friends. Further, they were *least* likely to be church members or to attend church services, or to belong to and participate in formal organizations or groups. Obviously, the cumulative consequences of these conditions would lead to an insufficient amount of stimulating and rewarding social interaction. Younger male survivors, on the other hand, usually are able to avoid these problems through remarriage.

Remarriage and Mortality Risk

Remarriage may, in fact, have life-extending potentialities. For example, in the study just cited, in addition to finding that for both sexes mortality rates were significantly higher for those who lived alone, it also revealed that, for most age ranges, the death rates among remarried widowers were significantly *lower* than those among married males. Unfortunately, the causes for these differences have not been pinpointed. Some support was found for both the *selectivity hypothesis*, which argues that the healthy remarry and the sick do not, as well as for the *social support network hypothesis,* which argues that remarriage provides conditions for care and support that are effective in ameliorating the effects of bereavement and thereby reducing mortality risk. As the authors put it, "the continual availability of even one person for conversation and assistance in an emergency may be even more effective that a large number of friends or relatives who visit less frequently."[225]

Social Support. While we know that social support may play a major role in achieving a longer and healthier life, we don't know exactly how it operates to protect us against stress and other hazards. The literature reveals many diverse ways of defining and measuring the dimensions of social support. In attempting to develop more precise definitions of this concept researchers have focused on some its major indicators. One such indicator is the level of *social integration*—the degree to which a person has regular access to the potential sources of support or is isolated from them. It has been found that persons high on measures of social integration exhibit better mental and physical health and greater longevity than those who are lower on such measures. Social support has the potential to promote health and well-being in several ways, including meeting our basic needs for meaningful relationships, reducing or mitigating our exposure to stress and other health hazards at work or elsewhere, and, where exposure to stress cannot be avoided, buffering its impact on health. In short, the active presence of others, especially familiar others, strengthens one's ability to survive.[226] Social relationships and activity can enhance the quality as well as the quantity of life. Therefore, specification of the kinds of social networks that are the most beneficial has become an important scientific objective. Hopefully, in the future, measures will be available which allow people to determine not only if they are getting enough, but also the right kinds of support to reap its benefits.[227]

The Gender Differential: Women and Long Life

It has long been known that sex differences in longevity consistently favor females. This is true in this country and other parts of the world. A perusal of the leading causes of death in the United States quickly reveals that all of them kill more men than women. For example, heart disease, lung cancer, homicide, cirrhosis of the liver, and pneumonia, each leads to the demise of men at roughly twice the rate for women. Some of this gender difference may be attributed to the greater damage that men inflict upon themselves—they smoke and drink more than women and take many more life-threatening chances. Moreover, compared to women, men are murdered (typically by other men) three times as often, commit suicide at a higher rate, experience more than twice as many fatal automobile accidents, and are more likely to be involved in alcohol-related fatalities. Even when these behavioral differences are taken into account, however, the longevity advantage of women still remains, suggesting that they may be born with a biological advantage which makes them less vulnerable to life-threatening diseases.

Scientists disagree as to the relative weights that should be given to the biological and behavioral factors. They generally agree, however, that a full explanation of gender mortality differences requires taking into account both the *biogenic* and the *psychosocial* factors that influence life expectancy. Moreover, there is little question that a significant portion of the higher death rates among men is related to the lethal aspects of a wide range of behaviors associated with traditional male role expectations.[228] These cultural expectations often lead to risky and destructive behavioral patterns, often motivated by the desire prove one's masculinity. It may be that in order to enhance their survival potential, men may have to give up a strict adherence to traditional male stereotypes. "It is time that men especially begin to comprehend that the price paid for belief in the male role is a shorter life expectancy. The male sex role will become less hazardous to our health only insofar as it ceases to be defined as opposite to the female role, and comes to be defined as one genuinely human way to live" (p. 83).

Interestingly, women appear to be more vulnerable to everyday types of sicknesses and pain. Compared to men, they visit physicians more often, take more prescription and nonprescription drugs, spend more days bedridden when ill, suffer from arthritis, bunions, bladder infection, corns, hemorrhoids, menstrual distress, migraine headaches, and varicose veins. As the author from whom we draw these comparisons so aptly put it: "Meanwhile men get heart attacks and strokes. Women are sick, but men are dead."[229] He also notes, however, that in recent decades lifestyle changes on the part of men have narrowed the health gap between the sexes. Hence, the life-expectancy advantage of women has been narrowing. Indeed, if current trends continue, the existing gap in longevity will disappear around 2040 in the United States.[230] Men are smoking and drinking less, and improving their dietary habits. Some argue that this narrowing of the longevity gap reflects the fact that women have suffered a decline in lifetime health from assuming more and more behavioral characteristics of men. Perhaps a more reasonable conclusion would be that men are adopting life-saving behavioral characteristics long associated with women. In any event, the fact remains that women in general, and wives in particular, continue to exhibit a greater probability of outliving their male counterparts.

Marrying a Younger Woman. The greater longevity of wives is one of the major factors underlying the growing population of widows in the United States. For several decades now, the ratio of widows to widowers has steadily widened. For example, in 1930, widows outnumbered their male counterparts by roughly two to one, whereas, today, that ratio has increased to more than four to one.[231] One way that husbands can decrease this greater mortality risk, vis a vis wives, is to marry a younger woman. It has been shown that marriage to a younger wife is significantly related to husband's longevity.[232] One team of analysts[233] examined national data and discovered significant mortality differentials for husbands married to younger and older wives. They found that men married to younger women have a lower risk of dying than men married to women of the same age or older.

At least two possible alternative hypotheses have been advanced by researchers for the conclusion that marriage to a younger woman enhances the survivorship probabilities of men. One stresses the *premarital selection factor*, that is, that healthier, wealthier, or more vigorous men select, or are selected by, younger women. The other emphasizes the influence of *postmarital personal interactions*, that is, being married to a younger woman is somehow psychologically, physiologically, or socially beneficial. Unfortunately, the nature of the data precluded a direct test of either of these alternatives.

We have seen evidence that remarriage has life-extension potential, especially for males. In the case of *older men*, however, courtship opportunities may be extremely limited unless they have unusual resources. Even with such resources, and even if the older person is successful in locating a potential mate, he may still have to overcome a lingering cultural bias in American society that sometimes discourages such unions. Thus, for example, the older widower contemplating remarriage often discovers that

> A barrier has been erected between what he wishes to do and what society expects him to do. His friends, his children, and the community at large rise up and condemn his remarriage. He is regarded as "too old for that." The wagging fingers, the knowing smiles, the raised eyebrows and the cruel tongues are set in motion. Marriage is for the young in age, not the young in heart[234] (p. 6).

Such attitudes and negative sanctions can effectively restrain an individual from remarrying and even force the couple to marry in secret. McKain found that elderly couples who marry in spite of family and community pressure sometimes do so by crossing state lines in order to avoid public opinion and censure. It is assumed that in the many years since his study was completed that such attitudes have become more tolerant with a concomitant diminution of biases toward marriages among older persons.

The Power of Meaningful Human Contacts

The preceding pages have ranged over a variety of social situations and relationships that influence our survival. From that discussion, one major conclusion emerges: The maintenance of meaningful human contacts somehow prevents illness and leads to life-extension. The absence or loss of such relationships, on the other hand, can be life-threatening. It is ironic, therefore, that American society so strongly encourages individualism and independence (for instance, "Stand on your own two feet," "Make it on your own," and "Do your own thing"), especially among its young. While such attributes are laudable and produce many positive outcomes for the individual, they also have certain disadvantages.

Living Alone. While much is made of the single lifestyle and its advantages, the fact is that people who live alone, regardless of age or sex, experience significantly higher death rates than those who are married or live with others. This is also the case for major causes of premature death, such as heart disease, automobile accidents, lung cancer, suicide, cirrhosis of the liver, and stroke[235],[236] For example, researchers at three New York hospitals tracked patients who had survived a heart attack to determine whether their living arrangements affected their health. They found that patients who lived alone were nearly twice as likely at those with companions to have another attack—or die from one—within six months. None of the known risk factors for a second heart attack—advanced age, lower socioeconomic status, or severe heart damage—accounted for the ill health of the subjects who lived by themselves.[237] The evidence strongly suggests that a major contributing factor is isolation and associated loneliness, leading to the conclusion that:

> ...enduring human relationships—between children and parents, among friends, and, most importantly, between husbands and wives—are essential prerequisites for emotional and physical well-being. In fact, people without such intimate, long-lasting ties are more likely to suffer disabling disease and even premature death.[238]

A single lifestyle correlates with serious medical problems, whereas a stable, satisfactory marriage, or even living together, decreases the probability of such occurrences. A review of more than 130 empirical studies that related marital status to various well-being indices, including alcoholism, suicide, morbidity and mortality, schizophrenia or other psychiatric problems, and self-reports of happiness revealed a consistent pattern: "Married individuals, especially married men, experience less stress and emotional pathology than their unmarried counterparts." Moreover, the accumulated evidence strongly supports the *protection\support hypothesis*, which posits that the married "experience less physical and emotional pathology than the unmarried because they have continuous companionship with a spouse who provides interpersonal closeness, emotional gratification, and support in dealing with daily stress."[239]

It is important to point out that nonmarried status, by itself, does not diminish life chances. If single people, especially the separated, divorced, and widowed, develop and maintain meaningful relationships, the positive quality of those relationships will be more influential than the mere fact that they are single. Nor is the experience of living alone, *per se*, necessarily detrimental to one's social or psychological well-being. Persons living by themselves often compensate for their "aloneness" by having greater contact with others outside the household. Moreover, living alone, "rather than being a catastrophic situation into which persons are forced against their will, appears to be an arrangement of choice in many instances, or at least one which is readily adjusted to, leaving undisturbed one's relative satisfaction with life."[240] Given the fact that for a variety of reasons the proportion of people living alone in the United States has dramatically increased in recent decades, it is important to recognize that such living arrangements do not preclude sustaining close relationships with others, and with persons who can provide close emotional support for problems of daily living. In sociological terms, it does not necessarily prevent one's ability to develop and maintain a healthy level of social integration, for example, by being embedded in neighborhood and friendship networks which promote personal well-being.[241]

Significant Others and Survival. The evidence cited in the previous pages points to the crucial role and, indeed, the necessity of *significant others* in our lives.[242] Apparently such people help directly in our efforts to cope with the stresses of daily living. It also suggests that the choice to live alone may inadvertently lead to increased vulnerability to serious medical and emotional problems. For example, the single, widowed, and divorced visit their physicians nearly twice as often as married persons; and they remain in hospitals nearly twice as long for similar medical problems. Thus, continuous and stable human intimacy seems to be an essential ingredient for the maintenance of good health.

An appreciation of the importance of human love, one of "the most vital of human behaviors," along with tenderness, compassion, caring, sharing, relating, and companionship, seems to be absent from many lives.[243] The risks some people take in failing to recognize and fulfill these basic needs may ultimately result in illness or premature demise. Admittedly, avoiding loneliness is not easy in our society, which fosters uprootedness and stresses the importance of making it on one's own. However, a lifelong effort to establish and maintain a network or intimate, meaningful social ties appears essential to our survival. Luciano de Crescenzo perhaps put it most eloquently: "We are each of us angels with only one wing. And we can only fly embracing each other."

8

Modifying Habits: Reducing Risks

The probability of staying alive and well is partly dependent on the degree to which a person actively pursues the goals of self-knowledge and self-control. Achievement of these goals hinges on how diligently one practices "selfwatching," a conscious program of systematic self-surveillance in order to understand and then change behavior which can be life-threatening.[244] This effort includes a preventive orientation, one designed to alter or halt dangerous habits and to minimize their associated risks. However, modifying lifetime practices requires a high degree of commitment, motivation, *and* a plan of action, in order to avoid *relapses*. Even addictions or compulsions, which are basically strong habits, often can be successfully modified or even unlearned if proper strategies are consistently followed. Again, attitudes are critical:

> attitudes play perhaps the most central role in fitness; without your sincere desire to be well and fit, all else is lost and unattainable. This attitude is your willingness to apply the knowledge that comes from medical advances, by actively intervening against known risk factors, by seeking help whenever necessary to change deleterious behavior at any age, and through your commitment to participate actively in health monitoring.[245]

Everyone has habits, some of which are beneficial, and the majority of which are harmless. However, when certain habits get out of control and become strongly resistant to change they become compulsions, and as such, they can disrupt daily living, damage relationships, and destroy health.[246] Hodgson and Miller offer several steps designed to strengthen self-control skills. The first technique is that of *self-observation*, and involves keeping a diary in which the person notes all instances of the targeted behavior which occur during the day. The time of day, the antecedent or preceding behaviors, the actual behavior, and its consequences are all recorded. These exercises will help to identify situations in which the unwanted activity is most likely to occur. It is more effective to make the diary entry *before* initiating the behavior in order to sensitize one to what is taking place. The more specific the information which is recorded, the more effective this technique seems to be in modifying behavior.[247]

The second technique is that of *self-management*. After the diary has been analyzed, the specific circumstances which trigger the targeted behavior can be identified. Self-management is a conscious attempt to control behavior through several strategies, the first of which involves *rearranging the environment*.[248] Place/ time associations which provoke habits can be replaced. If a smoker always has a cigarette with a cup of coffee, replacing the coffee with another beverage may reduce the urge to smoke. A person can rearrange the circumstances which give rise to the problematic behavior. A second strategy is that of *modifying the consequences* of a behavior. This relates to rewards or punishment for positive or negative behavior. These sanctions must take place soon after the action has occurred to be effective. Research suggests that it is important to reward an ongoing pattern of behavior rather than only the attainment of a goal.[249] Punishment should be used only in combination with rewards to be the most constructive. *Thought control* is another self-management strategy. Here, thinking rather than behavior is being modified. The goal is to improve a person's perspective by encouraging him or her to invoke positive rather than negative thoughts. Positive thoughts are scheduled to occur just before some common behavior. The person is instructed to think a positive thought related to the behavior problem every time he sits down or answers the phone. The last self-management strategy involves *restraint*. Here the person is instructed to delay acting on temptation for at least ten minutes. This allows time for the cravings to subside, for a more logical decision to be made, and for consideration of the long term consequences of giving in to the craving.

The third self-watching technique is to *face up to reality*. A person simply cannot avoid temptation for his entire life. This technique involves deliberately exposing oneself to a temptation and then refrain from giving in to it. This will make it easier to resist giving in the next time. With repeated practice, the power of the temptation should gradually diminish. It is best to begin with the minor and least dangerous enticements, and then gradually expose oneself to increasingly greater allurements as the lesser ones are conquered.

Not all habitual behavior is, of course, detrimental to our health and welfare. Much of it is adaptive and helps ensure survival, for example, when we automatically look both ways before crossing a street or highway. Habits are learned, automatic behaviors that often provide immediate pleasure and comfort. Others, however, while still giving immediate satisfaction, can nonetheless have long-term negative consequences. "Those habits most firmly associated with either strong feelings of pleasure or with the avoidance of distress are the most likely to develop into compulsions which damage the quality of our lives."[250] As such they are especially difficult to alter or terminate because they have become solidly entrenched through the processes of positive or negative reinforcement. Hence, they carry with them a high potential for human suffering. The person attempting to eliminate strongly routinized behavioral patterns often finds that under stress he or she will automatically revert to them. Such *habit relapses* are very common. Some estimate that four-fifths of those who try to break a habit will relapse within three months.[251]

Self-Help and Support Groups

Despite the difficulties just noted, it appears that under proper regimens and conditions, bad habits can be permanently abandoned. Many people are, in fact, able to "kick the habit" on their own through sheer determination. Indeed, one student of addictions contends that *self-reliance* is the best means for getting rid of unhealthy habits; that depending on others to cure you usually does not work.[252] He argues that encouraging people to rely upon others to correct their bad habits and addictions allows them to avoid responsibility for their behavior. His philosophy of self-cure, which many accept, "translates into three components necessary for change: an urge to quit, the belief that you *can* quit and the realization that *you* must quit—no one can do it for you." Often, however, the exertion of will power alone, the "pulling yourself up by your own bootstraps," approach, is insufficient to do the job. Many believe a greater degree of success can be achieved by combining positive motivation and self-mastery techniques with participation in support groups, such as Alcoholics Anonymous, Smokenders, and Weightwatchers.

Support groups organized to meet a variety of needs have proliferated across the country. Hundreds of counseling organizations and self-help groups have emerged in response to the growing interest in death and dying issues. Much of the impetus for the creation of these groups came from widows and widowers seeking information and assistance that would help them get through the bereavement process and make a healthy recovery from the loss of a mate. Today, several cities have networks of bereavement counseling centers, some of them affiliated with national organizations such as the Widowed Persons Service, an arm of the National Retired Teachers Association. Active involvement in such groups may have survival benefits. For instance, a decade long study found that terminally ill cancer patients who participated in weekly support-group meetings while receiving treatment lived nearly twice as long as those given only medical care.[253]

Self-help support groups, organized to meet an ever-widening range of needs, dramatically have increased and now involve millions of Americans meeting on a weekly or monthly basis every year. Their growth, in fact, has been phenomenal and is reflected in the establishment of numerous local and national self-help clearinghouse offices across the nation. Volunteers staff them and assist people in locating a desired support group to address their particular problem.

Support groups are based upon the premise that most people need external assistance to break their harmful habits. They differ from group psychiatry therapy in that they are composed entirely of peers. The goal of the group is to provide emotional and social support to members with similar problems. The success rate reported by self-help groups has been encouraging. However, there is some controversy over the rate of recidivism among people attempting to change or eliminate bad habits. Hodgson and Miller, for example, cite a study which found that about two-thirds of smokers, alcoholics and drug addicts repeat their behaviors again within three months of their initial resolve to change. On the other hand, those who manage to abstain during the first three to six months have an excellent chance of avoiding relapse. Others claim that nine out of ten dieters regain all the weight they lose, and that over eighty percent of all those who quit smoking eventually light up again. Still others argue that statistics are misleading because they are based primarily upon therapy/client group populations. Schachter studied two groups who had not sought professional help and found that more than sixty percent of the smokers who tried to quit and the over-eaters who tried to lose weight reported success.[254]

Relapse Prevention

We earlier discussed *selfwatching*, a holistic monitoring technique to enhance people's lives by reducing or eliminating complex habits or addictions. A related self-management program is called *relapse prevention*. This is particularly useful in helping people to mediate habitual risk behavior. It is not a tool which can be used to directly effect a change in behavior. Instead, it assists people in maintaining their new, healthier, and less hazardous life-styles. Habit breaking can be accomplished through a variety of tactics. However, once the behavior has been initially modified, the arduous task of maintenance ensues.

Relapse prevention assists in the maintenance of the new balanced life-style in a manner unlike some commonly accepted programs. This is because it is based on a different philosophy of habitual behavior. The *model of relapse prevention* builds from the belief that habits are learned, and are reinforced through positive stimuli. This is unlike the *disease model*, which essentially assumes individuals cannot help themselves, or a related *moral model*, which blames the victim for initially taking up the habit. Together they give rise to a *control paradox*. They assume that once the habit is initiated that the victim is no longer in control of his own behavior. If a person attempts to quit the habit and fails, these models deem that loss of control is a failure on the part of the individual, who is assumed not to have control in the first place! In contrast, in the relapse prevention model nobody is blamed for the development of the habitual behavior. Secondly, once a person quits the habit, he is *expected* to experience lapses. Furthermore, recurrences are not viewed as failures but rather as beneficial learning experiences. In this perspective, because it is a learning experience, each relapse serves to deter further repetitions. Hence, recurrences are expected to decline as people move away from the time they first attempted to quit. Under the disease model, however, as people backslide, they begin to believe that they are out of control. Because they feel that there is nothing they can do to help themselves, repetitions occur more frequently as people move away from the experience which initially caused them to abstain from the unwholesome behavior.

Each person is his own agent of change under the optimistic relapse prevention model—habits do not control people, people control habits. The goal of this approach is self-determination through self-control. However, to accomplish this goal, a person needs to be educated about how to handle the crises of relapses. Often the initiation of this self-management program comes from support systems which the habit victim seeks out or is placed into for help. The evidence suggests that the greatest probability of success derives from a combination of individual initiative and group support offered by self-help organizations. In order to abandon permanently a bad habit one also has to simultaneously unlearn certain behaviors and replace them with others that also provide gratification. This is a difficult task, but the fact that many people succeed means that with practice and persistence it can be accomplished.

Several strategies have been offered by successful quitters for dealing with problem habits, including (1) planning ahead as to what to do when periodic relapse urges occur, for example, going for a walk, gardening, talking with a friend; (2) substituting activities that provide similar, satisfying results and meet the emotional needs that the bad habits did, for example, exercise programs, dancing; (3) seeking assistance from family and friends as well as support groups, such as Alcoholic Anonymous, Weight Watchers); (4) avoiding high-risk situations, for instance, pass up tempting social situations to avoid overeating); (5) setting realistic goals which are achievable, for example, a short-term goal of one week of abstinence from hard liquor or desserts); (6) rewarding yourself for sticking with your regimen, for example, buy yourself a new skirt. Rewards help reinforce the motivation or will power to continue the regimen; (7) retaining an honest perspective with respect to your motivations and behavior, for example, denying that you have arranged tempting conditions which will lead to relapse, like purchasing a bottle of whiskey by rationalizing that it is necessary in case company should drop in); (8) should a relapse occur, taking action to resist a repetition, for example, giving in to the urge to smoke should immediately be followed by a realization of the negative consequences of continuing, analyzing what triggered the relapse, and moving to avoid similar conditions. There are no "quick fixes" in getting rid of compulsive bad habits. A person has to be strongly inspired to get rid of them, and has to learn which strategies work best to accomplish this. A combination of patience and persistence, with an eye toward long-term results, is essential.[255]

Reducing Risks: The Health Professionals

Health professionals encounter difficulties in getting people to change life-threatening habits in order to reduce the risks of illness and premature mortality. They know, for example, that it is unrealistic to expect individuals to change their behavior simply by appealing to their sense of personal responsibility. They also know that patients exhibit differential responses to techniques designed to enhance compliance.[256] Hence, while at first they may attempt to apply general principles of effecting change, often they have to develop educational programming which takes into account the principle of "different strokes for different folks." Programs designed to accommodate specific types of individuals, especially those who fall into hard to reach or high-risk groups, are particularly expensive, since they often require counseling sessions, home visits, and the like to reinforce a preventive health care regimen.

The Role of Values. Many argue that the elimination of damaging habits and the reduction of health risks can be achieved *only* when the person becomes *personally* sensitive to the risk.[257] The patient who is told by his dentist that the black spot on his palate is a precancerous sign, and that he should see a patholo-gist immediately, is apt to take notice! If the pathologist strongly suggests that he give up his heavy pipe smoking, and shows him pictures of the cancerous mouths of those who did not follow this recommendation, he might just give the habit up. For some people, this combination of education and frightening revelation works. For others, the lesson is only short-lived, and they eventually return to their prior pattern of self-inflicted injury (Many automobile drivers have been ticketed for speeding, fined, and sent to driver school. Yet they continue to speed).

A different approach to such personalization is for the health professional to ascertain what the individual values most and then to focus behaviors and educa-tion relative to those values. A person may be more receptive to a discussion of eliminating a particular activity when he recognizes that it threatens that which he values most. Allowing people to choose risks related to what they value most may achieve greater compliance. A discussion of this type is more likely to pro-vide a positive climate between the individual and the health care provider.

This approach is of particular interest to those concerned with health behav-iors because such actions frequently involve the conflict of choosing between unhealthy acts, which may appear to be glamorous or exciting, and healthier acts, which may require more persistent effort. Its been shown that the values a person holds can be a predictor of behavior, and when *value confrontation* occurs, the individual can modify his value system and achieve behavioral changes.[258] This confrontation technique involves raising the persons's awareness of the contradic-tions among his or her self-concepts, values, and behavior. It then seeks to achieve those changes necessary to restore consistency among them. The signifi-cance of a value is determined by its relation to other values. Hence, one needs to look at the extent to which someone values health in relation to other values, rather than the value of health as an absolute. This is especially important if the acts in question are in competition with other behaviors related to more central values.[259]

Summary

Not infrequently, people simply outgrow earlier "cravings" and bad habits over time and with increasing maturity.[260] For some persons, eliminating bad health habits is accomplished with relative ease, and they are able to do so on their own. For others, it become more of a struggle, and they must rely on the help of family and friends. For those whose habits have become addictions and compulsions, the assistance of health providers and educators, as well as support groups may be essential to sustain the kinds of permanent changes in lifestyle that are required. For those who believe that the individual must take primary responsibility for this curative process, the succinct advice by Peele regarding the basic steps for working one's way out of an addiction may prove helpful: "find a superior alternative to the habit you want to break; find people who can help you puncture your complacent defenses; change whatever you need in your life to accommodate your new, healthier habits; celebrate your new, nonaddicted image whenever you can."[261]

9

The Societal Context of Survival: Part 1

We have noted that heredity, personal habits, reaction to stress, and social support networks are key dimensions of understanding how individuals remain healthy and alive. However, staying alive is also highly dependent on conditions and events which characterize the larger social worlds in which we live. In this chapter we concentrate on some of the salient societal and socio-demographic influences that affect life chances in the United States. These chances vary by regional patterns as well as by an array of other sociocultural dimensions of our society. For example, residing in a region where mining is a major activity can have deleterious consequences for one's health and longevity. Not only are death rates higher in such areas, but this holds true for the residents whether they work in the mines or not. Even women who do not work in mines suffer higher death rates than females in non-mining areas. This is probably due to a combination of sociocultural factors, exposure to mining waste products, and perhaps selective out-migration of hardier, stronger people.[262]

Even regional patterns, however, evidence the ubiquitous influence of lifestyle factors. A well known example is Fuchs's comparison of the health differences between Nevada and Utah.[263] These contiguous states had about the same levels of income and medical care, and were similar in many other respects—schooling, degree of urbanization, climate, even number of physicians and hospital beds. But the levels of health for their respective populations were dramatically different. "The inhabitants of Utah are among the healthiest individuals in the United States, while the residents of Nevada are at the opposite end of the spectrum." For example, the infant mortality rate was about 40 percent higher in Nevada, and its adult death rate was 40 to 50 percent higher than Utah. Fuchs finds the explanation for these hugh differences in the contrasting lifestyles of the residents. Utah is a state dominated by its large Mormon population. They avoid the use of tobacco or alcohol and in general lead stable, quite lives. In contrast, Nevada residents exhibit high rates of cigarette and alcohol consumption, as well as much greater levels of marital and geographical instability. For example, at the time of the study more than 60 percent of Utah's residents 20 years of age or older were native-born, compared to only 10 percent in Nevada. In other words, its population consisted predominantly of recent immigrants, many coming because of the state's permissive mores. The differences in marital status were equally significant. Over one-fifth of the males between the ages of 35-64 living in Nevada at the time were single, widowed, divorced, or separated from their spouses and, among married couples, over a third had been previously widowed or divorced. The comparable figures were only half as large for Utah residents. Clearly, such differences cannot be explained by such factors as the availability of medical care or income, and the evidence strongly points to the significant role played by lifestyle variations between residents of these two states.

Low Status and Early Death

Race and social class especially influence one's potential for living because of society's differential sensitivity to members of those groups. The two characteristics are often linked. In this connection racial differences in mortality are particularly revealing. The average life expectancy of whites is five to seven years longer than blacks. This racial disparity is closely correlated to socioeconomic factors which, in turn, affect the survival rates of all racial groups. Evidence in this country and many others, "points consistently to the social inequality of death for members of different social strata."[264]

Kidney transplant patients provide a clear illustration of the racial inequality with respect to access to life-saving facilities. Several studies have showed that in the United States white men are twice as likely to get new kidneys as blacks of either sex and a third more likely than white women. It appears this discrepancy remains even when patients are from comparable socioeconomic groups. This racial disparity exists despite the fact that blacks have three times the rate of kidney failure as whites. It remains even though for decades the federal government has attempted to remove the economic barriers to such operations by absorbing the majority of the costs. The government also pays the full costs of kidney dialysis, whereby a machine cleanses the blood in place of the patient's failed kidneys. How does one account for the racial imbalance in kidney transplants? Some bioethicists have suggested that one factor may be an unconscious bias on the part of physicians who refer such patients to transplant centers, feeling that "people who are richer, have jobs, and are more assertive, will do better as transplant recipients than people who are poor, unemployed, and passive."[265] Documenting such factors is extremely difficult, but there is little question that blacks have less access to health services in general than do whites.

The area of heart transplants similarly reveals the influence of racial and socioeconomic factors on life chances. Researchers have detected *queue jumping* in organ transplantation. This occurs when candidates less likely to benefit from transplants, because of underlying disease or other contra-indications, receive organs over persons deemed more likely to benefit. The Agency for Health Care Policy found that higher-income patients or those with private insurance were twice as likely to receive heart transplants despite contra-indications, as were poorer, non-privately insured patients with no contra-indications.[266]

The Maldistribution of Risk. Federal data has consistently revealed that the poor are at a clear disadvantage with respect to health status. Poor adults are "more likely than adults who were not poor to be in fair or poor health."[267] In addition to the differential access to medical treatment, this disadvantage constitutes what Baker terms the **maldistribution of risk.** She notes that the loss of potential years of life is much greater for traumatic events (injuries) than for any disease. However, such events are distributed unequally among our population. "There are distinct differences in death rates and injury rates among various racial groups; in each group, people of low economic status are especially disadvantaged."[268] She presents several examples of this maldistribution of risk. With respect to race, for instance, black males are at much greater risk for becoming victims of homicide than other groups. In terms of age and gender differences, the risks of suicide are much higher among elderly males compared to elderly females. Teenagers and young adults are much more susceptible to fatal motor vehicle crashes, especially those involving alcohol, than other age groups. It turns out that motor vehicle fatalities and death from other causes of injury are particularly prominent in rural areas. There are even regional differences in death rates from house fires; they are highest in the Southeast where "highly flammable homes, noncentral heating sources, and great distances from fire-fighting equipment all contribute to the hazard of death by conflagration." (p. 140).

It is generally assumed that with proper precautions and interventions, many of these deaths from unintentional injuries would not have occurred. However, Baker argues that until death rates from causes which disproportionaly affect specific groups are redefined as important public health problems, little change will occur, since the people involved generally lack the requisite political power to bring about change on their own.

A contrasting outcome results when the larger public is exposed to random risks, in which case anyone could be affected. The Tylenol scare that took place not too long ago is illustrative. When several people suddenly died of Tylenol poisoning, widespread public concern quickly led to a consensus that something must be done, and within a relatively short time the manufacturer introduced tamper-proof packaging to protect all users. AIDS provides another example. As long as its victims were defined as members of a despised minority, the problem was given insufficient attention. Only when AIDS spread to other populations, and the citizenry aroused, did it get defined as a public health problem, and given national attention and action. In summary, unless the larger public feels vulnerable, calls for action on the part of the affected populations to reduce their risks may go unheeded.

The Urban Environment: Staying Alive in the City

Additional support for the *social inequality hypothesis* comes from a study of Columbus, Ohio, which found that social status levels and, more importantly, housing conditions affected the death rate.[269] There are also risk aspects of urban life in general that affect our potential for living. People residing in the central or inner cores of our large cities are especially vulnerable to a host of social, economic, educational, and nutritional deficiencies, often reflected in high crime rates, which undermine their life chances. The negative consequences of urban life, especially as they relate to health and longevity, know no national boundaries. For example, the extremely high rate of heart disease in Moscow proper has been linked to smoking, alcoholism, and stress resulting from crowded urban living environments.[270] In America, it has been found that poor blacks of Detroit who live in areas of high unemployment, crime and violence, and poor housing also exhibit a high incidence of hypertension. In addition, the highest mortality rates in Boston occur in the black ghetto as well as in working-class areas of whites. Mortality rates in these "death zones" are elevated both for hypertension-related ailments like stroke and for all other causes of death.[271]

Some of the hazardous aspects of urban life are beyond the direct control of the individual. While one may write Congress, for example, to enact new anti-pollution laws, the more immediate presence of that pollution is beyond the control of the individual (except insofar as one is fortunate enough to be able to relocate to a less polluted environment). Nevertheless, some sense of personal control is an essential element of coping with city life. It's been found, for example, that excessive noise pollution was not so negative when people had the option of "turning-off" that noise. Even when this option is never exercised, the knowledge that one could choose to do so was often sufficient to alleviate much of its intrusive impact.[272]

Urbanites can and often do implement a range of strategies to gain some control over their surroundings. They can plan alternate routes home to avoid delays from accidents; they can have preplanned strategies to put into place on days of snowstorms when transportation is problematic; they can choose indoor exercise activities on days of high air pollution. The important thing is to plan a variety of options for diverse situations. Such planning enables a person to anticipate stressful and physically damaging situations and actively lessen their impact.

Emphasizing the strains of city living often leads to an idyllic view of life in the country—an abundance of clean air, friendly neighbors, peaceful solitude, etc. This is far from true. Rural life, it turns out, has its own set of risks and stresses, especially if one is trying to work the land. Such labor can be tremendously exhausting. Farmers can rarely afford to stay sick or take vacations. They have to cope with isolation, economic problems, equipment breakdowns, sick animals, crop failures, and having to travel miles to stores or medical facilities. Hence, the stresses of rural living can cause many familiar problems—mental illness, divorce, even suicide. There has been a slow but growing recognition that stress-management programs are also needed by those who choose to live "down on the farm."

Technological and Social Change

The demographic and geographic dimensions of mortality do not, of course, fully characterize the interplay between societal forces and survival capability. Changes on the societal level have significant consequences for the length and quality of life. The Industrial Revolution and urbanization in America and Western Europe were corollaries to an increase in longevity and standard of living. The accompanying decline in birth rates, for example, diminished one of the chief threats to women since high numbers of pregnancies increase their chances of premature death. By lowering the growth of population, industrialization and technological development allowed the benefits of modernization to be shared more abundantly than if birth rates had remained high.

Relatively simple technological innovations can have far-reaching effects on our ability to stay alive, if they can be accepted by the general population. For example, in an earlier chapter we noted that the automobile industry long possessed an involuntary device to provide safety for American drivers—the air bag. While industry representatives agreed that automatically inflated air bags would reduce the risks of an accidental death, for years they resisted installing them as standard equipment. They lobbied against proposed legislation to make this involuntary device mandatory on all cars. Generally, they argued that the installation and maintenance is cost prohibitive and would affect sales. Eventually, of course, they were mandated to install air bags in all cars, and their earlier negative prognostications failed to materialize. This long-standing controversy over air bags brings into sharp focus the ever present conflict in other arenas between economic values and those placed upon preserving human life.

High-Risk Technologies. The rapid evolution of complex and high-risk technologies in recent decades has brought with it a heightened catastrophic potential. Examples of this include nuclear power plants, nuclear weapons systems, ships, trucks, or trains carrying highly toxic or explosive cargoes, and the accumulation of petrochemical wastes and toxic discharges. These and other risky enterprises have the ability to cripple, shorten the lives of, or actually to kill large numbers of people in a single incident. The industrial chemical disaster at the Union Carbide pesticide plant on the outskirts of Bhopal, India in 1984, and the 1986 nuclear accident at Chernobyl, in the then Soviet Union, the dire effects of which are still being felt today twenty years later, are illustrative. Both tragedies killed large numbers of people and left lingering, long-term health problems for survivors. Both vividly demonstrated the life-threatening potential of modern industrial enterprises, even when safety precautions have been taken. The Bhopal disaster resulted from the release of *methyl isocyanate*, a colorless liquid chemical compound which transforms into a gas at high temperatures. The plants automatic safety systems failed to prevent the deadly gas from escaping into the community. Indeed, other major industrial accidents associated with the manufacture and storage of sophisticated chemicals have occurred in several countries, despite safety precautions.

Perrow[273] has argued that, no matter how effective conventional safety devices are, a majority of high-risk systems have some special characteristics, beyond their toxic or genetic dangers, that make accidents in them inevitable, even "normal." This has to do with the way failures can interact and the way systems are tied together. One system characteristic which leads to inevitable accidents are automatic controls. Not all controls can be operated by humans. Some operations require precise timing or quick execution. In such situations automatic controls must be used. Because such controls can execute steps quickly, they are often difficult to stop. Instead of a human pressing a button to initiate each step in a series, automatic controls execute the steps immediately. Perrow refers to these types of systems as *tightly coupled*; there is no buffer or slack between steps A and

B. In tightly coupled systems failed parts cannot be isolated from other working parts, and it becomes impossible to keep production going safely. Unfortunately, many systems must be tightly coupled or they simply cannot operate. Thus, many accidents are not a result of operator error, planning error, or component failure. Rather, the complexity of the system itself is to blame for many accidents resulting in lost lives.

The widely publicized accident at the Three Mile Island nuclear plant in Pennsylvania in is another example of the catastrophic potential of complex technological systems. Indeed, because of the unusually high risk associated with such systems, Perrow suggests that some of them should be completely abandoned in favor of safer devices because:

> ...neither organizational structures nor technological innovations appear to make them any less prone to system accidents. In fact, these systems require organizational structures that have large internal contradictions, and technological fixes that only increase interactive complexity and tighten the coupling; they become still more prone to certain kinds of accidents...The odd term *normal accident* is meant to signal that, given the system characteristics, multiple and unexpected interactions of failures are inevitable. (p. 5).

We have already noted one such internal contradiction—the need to have tight coupling and automatic controls for the system to function properly, yet the same system may need loose coupling and operator controls to provide safety. A related contradiction surrounds the issue of system control. On the one hand, people managing subsystems will need great freedom and flexibility when unexpected accidents arise. Because the accidents will be unexpected no instructions or regulations will be in place to outline the best course of action. Unfortunately, the solution to the subsystem accident may adversely affect other subsystems. Thus central control is needed to assure that this does not occur. As the reader may have gathered by now, all this can rapidly get very complicated.

Another illustration of this complex interaction of technological systems is called *sequence jumping*. This occurs when an event in one linear system triggers the start of a separate linear sequence. Sequence jumping is often a result of physical proximity. For example, the crew of the Dauntless Colocotronis (an oil tanker) experienced a bizarre sequence jump when the tanker grazed the top of a sunken wreck in the Mississippi river, apparently because the depth charts were inaccurate. Though the graze was minor and barely noticed by the crew, it caused a small crack at the union of the tank and the boiler room. Oil seeped into the boiler room, became less viscous due to the heat in the room, and slid down a small shaft and into the engine room. The heat in the engine room caused the oil to evaporate and form an explosive gas. The gas was ignited by a spark in the room and an explosion occurred causing a fire. Perrow argues that this sort of sequence jumping is not at all predictable. And often, as in this example, no viable solution seems to exist. There is no where on the ship where the oil can be stored to guarantee that it never seeps into the engine room. The system of transporting oil in a marine vessel simply has inherent risks.

It is doubtful, of course, that any of these high-risk technologies will be eliminated in the near future. Therefore, to avoid life-threatening catastrophes or minimize their potential for causing widespread fatalities, better management of such enterprises must be developed and employed. This would include such improvements as better operator training, safer designs, more quality control, and more effective regulation. Without such improvements, the lives of large numbers of people will remain unnecessarily at risk. All too often, however, efforts to minimize or ameliorate the potentially life-threatening conditions are impeded by special interests more committed to maintaining a profit margin. Scientists are frequently dismayed by the harsh reality that the acceptability of risk is more often than not a political issue over which they have little influence.[274] These obstacles and conditions are apt to be with us for some time. As the remaining available fossil fuels are depleted, nuclear power will continue to grow steadily in importance as a major source of electricity.

Sophisticated technological and scientific changes can and have, of course, done much to eradicate threats to life. The advances of medicine have increased our well-being beyond levels ever thought possible. New medications, artificial hearts, organ transplants, and other advances help to promote both the quality of life and its duration. Interrelated with these advances, however, is the willingness of society to expend the monetary resources to make such technology accessible to the general population. The progress in curing heart disease perhaps best illustrates this. Several hundreds of millions of dollars a year are spent studying the cause, prevention and treatment of heart disease. The result has been a decline in the death rate from cardiovascular disease. Changes in lifestyles and risk factor reduction were major contributors to this decrease in mortality. New technology, improved pharmacology, better surgical techniques, and more effective medical management also played significant roles.[275]

The reduction in heart disease is attributable in part to changes in diets, treatment of hypertension, a decrease in smoking in middle-aged men, and an increase in exercise on a regular basis. It is also due to better treatment of coronary artery disease through the use of beta blocker compounds that reduce deaths from heart attacks, angioplasty to open clogged arteries, new enzymes to prevent irreversible heart muscle damage, the development of new machinery which detects areas starving for blood and oxygen, and the discovery of substances which seem to reduce greatly rejection in heart transplants. In the years ahead, we should see increased use of laser techniques to remove the placque that hardens arteries. We are already witnessing the development of new and more effective ways to lower cholesterol—a major modifiable risk factor for cardiovascular disease, along with high blood pressure and cigarette smoking. These are important developments with the potential for saving many lives. People with high blood pressure, for example, have three to four times the risk of developing coronary heart disease and as much as seven times the risk of a stroke as those with normal blood pressures.

The results, thus far, from these and related efforts have been pronounced and encouraging. In the last two decades, death rates have fallen 35 for diseases of the heart and blood vessels, for coronary heart disease, and for strokes. The average life expectancy continues to move upward—from about 70 years during the 1980's to over 75 today.

Unanticipated Consequences and Casualties

Medical innovations also open the door to unanticipated risks and human casualties. There has been a growing concern that while scientific advances have made medicine more effective, they also have created new dangers. It is now recognized that many of the new drugs which are able to control or cure previously fatal diseases also have the potential to injure or kill.[276] The most current example is the controversial arthritic painkiller Vioxx that was withdrawn from the market by its manufacturer after evidence that it could cause strokes and heart attacks. In other words, the modern drugs developed to prolong and improve life often can have side effects that destroy life. Surveys have shown that 10 to 18 percent (not an insignificant figure) of hospital patients develop reactions to drugs they receive. The mechanisms by which therapeutic drugs may cause death or disability include disturbance of body defense mechanisms, cell injury, imbalance of essential materials, genetic disturbances, chemical carcinogens, and change in microbial ecology. A widely known example here is *thalidomide*. As a sedative, this drug was to have enhanced the quality of life of pregnant women. Instead, it led to babies being born with severe limb distortions and other congenital anomalies. Although thalidomide was banned, another drug, *chloramphenicol*, is still in use. This antibiotic has the adverse effect of producing aplastic anemia, a suppression of bone marrow which proves fatal.

The use of drugs and other health remedies that have dangerous side effects are justified, in part, by the fact that the benefits outweigh the risks. In the case of thalidomide, of course, this was a false assertion. Since nearly all drugs carry side effects, banning all medication is not a logical solution. Proper testing and monitoring of drugs, on the other hand, is and should be a reasonable expectation. All too often, however, those responsible for such activity are delinquent in monitoring drugs and health aids—a problem we will examine in some detail a later chapter.

10

The Societal Context of Survival: Part 2

It took the Food and Drug Administration (FDA) years to put warning labels on very low-calorie, liquid-protein diet products. Yet it was common knowledge that many people had died from these diets; countless others suffered severe negative consequences. Long delays by the agency to ban drugs with adverse effects are not uncommon. Such delays are often a product of a complex and slow-moving bureaucracy, and the power of vested interests opposed to seeing products banned.

In recent years consumer groups and federal officials have questioned whether the Food and Drug Administration has, in fact, sufficient powers to protect the public from dangerous drugs and devices.[277] In the early 1990's several cases, involving *silicone* breast implants, the sleeping pill *Halcion*, and the sedative *Versed*, all suggested that the agency and the public are sometimes the last to learn of reports of dangerous side effects. Most people would be surprised to learn that this watch-dog agency does no testing itself. Rather, in making decisions it relies almost entirely on the test results submitted to it by manufacturers. Unfortunately, there is much evidence that at least some generic drug companies falsify test results or fail to report adverse reactions, or under-report side effects in order to get their products approved and marketed. Take, for example, the drug *Oraflex*. One executive of its manufacturer, Eli Lilly, testified that he had been aware of several overseas deaths linked to this arthritis drug before the FDA approved it, but chose not to inform the agency. The company pleaded guilty to 25 criminal misdemeanors in 1985, while its lawyer argued that it had acted "in good faith." *Sela*cryn, a drug for high blood pressure, was linked to over 30 deaths. Its maker, the Smith-Kline Beckman Corporation, pleaded guilty to not telling the FDA of foreign studies showing the danger. A German firm, Hoechst AG, was convicted because deaths resulting from its anti-depressant drug *Merita*l were not reported until long after it had marketed the drug in the United States in 1985. The Upjohn Company, the maker of Halcion, a leading sleep remedy, admitted having under-reported such side effects as paranoia and memory loss, discovered in its own 1973 study of the drug. Subsequently it forwarded corrected results to regulatory agencies and at the same time defended the study's original conclusions.

The list of known cases is uncomfortably long. In 1990 Congress reported that over half of the more than 200 new drugs marketed from the mid-seventies to the mid-eighties subsequently caused reactions severe enough to warrant label changes. Lobbied federal politicians have been reluctant to pass legislation which would give the FDA new powers to order off the market quickly products found to be dangerous and to fine companies that violate the rules. Few would disagree that: "Above all, there shines a clear need for basic ethics, the kind that deter companies from putting profits ahead of lives."[278]

Moreover, the FDA lacks the subpoena power, which nearly every other federal agency has, to obtain drug company documents when its suspicions are aroused. Even when people who have been harmed by drugs bring lawsuits, and their attorneys discover reports of side effects in the companies' files, the companies may refuse to settle the case unless all agree to the condition that the reports are sealed. Hence, years may pass before the agency gets to hear of vital information about hazards. In the case of silicone breast implants, the data that caused the commissioner of the FDA to ban them pending a review of their safety had long been known to the manufacturer. The details were disclosed to trial lawyers in the early 1980's, but the agency only learned of them in the early 1990's because they had been kept confidential under a court agreement. This case, as well as others, gives credence to the argument that this federal agency has limited abilities to assess the safety of drugs and devices accurately. Indeed, a highly critical 2006 government audit of this agency concluded that the "F.D.A. lacks clear and effective processes for making decisions about, and providing management oversight of issues involving the safety of popular medicines."[279]

Medical Technology: Potential Hazards.

Modern diagnostic procedures in medicine also entail unintended consequences that destroy life. These procedures involve the puncturing of arteries, veins, and other organs. They also include the catheterization of the urinary tract and blood vessels, as well as biopsies of a very delicate nature. The major hazards of these procedures are mechanical trauma to tissues or organs, anoxia of brain or heart, embolism, spread of tumor cells, infection, drug reactions, and disabling anxiety. For example, the technique of injecting contrast material into arteries (known as arteriography), has been widely adopted in recent years. But with this greater usage, "the dangers of anoxia and embolism are added to those of drug reaction and infection."[280] Unfortunately, the desire to prolong life, coupled with the pressure felt by many physicians to cover all the bases in order to avoid costly malpractice suits, results in more people being exposed to diagnostic and treatment procedures that are themselves life threatening.

Thus, changes in medical technology expose one to latent risks from the treatment itself. Moreover, the desire to extend longevity through technological innovations also leads to changes in the larger medical care delivery system. One major consequence has been a significant increase in medical care costs that are borne by individuals and the society-at-large. Illustrative here is the coronary-artery bypass operation. Years ago, this procedure was rarely used. Today, it has become the major surgical operation most frequently performed in the United States. Only those with adequate incomes or medical coverage are able to afford it. Congress and the nation are debating the morality and practicality of limiting medical costs with the possible consequences of restricting certain procedures only to those who have the financial resources to pay for them.

Other scientific applications affect our well-being in subtle and unexpected ways. A case in point is the massive amounts of antibiotics fed to farm animals in order to prevent the spread of bacterial infections.[281] One positive side effect of these drugs is that they somehow accelerate animal growth. However, evidence is accumulating which points to an unanticipated negative consequence and which links drug-saturated animal feed to human illness. The evidence, though far from definitive, suggests that animal antibiotics eventually produce antibiotic-resistant germs in animals, which are then transferred to humans through meat and poultry products.[282] Such germs were apparently responsible for a serious outbreak of gastrointestinal illness among a group of Minnesota residents. An investigative team of epidemiologists traced the bacterium to meat shipments from a South Dakota feed lot to supermarkets patronized by the victims. The feed lot had routinely added *chlorotetracycoline* to the animals' feed.

Not surprisingly, there is considerable debate over the human health hazards of antibiotic feed. Over the years several European countries have moved to limit the addition of certain drugs. In the United States, on the other hand, intensive lobbying by livestock breeders and pharmaceutical companies has blocked the passage of similar legislation in the Congress since it was first proposed by the Food and Drug Administration. It is worth noting that the pharmaceutical industry sells hundreds of millions of dollars worth of antibiotics to the feed industry each year.[283]

Dangerous Fish. Similar potential health hazards have been uncovered with respect to the fish we eat. The U.S. fishing industry hauls in billion pounds of fish annually. Over half the catch is consumed by humans; the rest ends up as pet food and other industrial products. American consumption per person has increase steadily. However, serious questions about the quality, wholesomeness, and safety of the fish we eat have been raised. Nearly half of the fish sampled (including shellfish) was contaminated by bacteria from human or animal feces. Some species examined were contaminated with PCB's and mercury, which can pose health hazards. Forty percent of the fish sampled exhibited bacteria counts indicating unacceptable spoilage levels. When bacteria counts hit 10 million or more, fish should be thrown away. Yet nearly 30 percent of the fish sample exceeded this level, and in nearly one-fourth, including most of the catfish, the counts surpassed the upper limits of the test method used.

The investigation also found that many retailers engaged in deceptive selling practices. Some would refer to their fish as fresh when in fact it had been frozen and then later thawed before being offered to the pubic. Indeed, as much as 15 days may have elapsed between the time the fish was caught and processed and the time it is purchased and eaten. Others, either deliberately or through ignorance, mislabeled the species they were selling. This was true of one-third of the fish sample, and it resulted not only in consumers eating fish different from what they thought they had purchased, but paying a higher price for it. This entire situation is compounded by the fact that, while close to two-thirds of America's fish are imported, officials are able to inspect less than 3 percent of it. They also manage to check less than a fifth of the thousands of seafood processing plants each year. Similarly inadequate meat-and-poultry inspection programs have long been a public health concern.

Those Harmful Stoves. A seemingly harmless trend in society can also affect our health, with potentially lethal consequences. With the petroleum crisis of the 1970s, Americans began to look for alternate forms of providing heat for homes. One of the most popular was the wood burning stove.[284] Approximately 20 percent of all homes now use wood burning for all or some of their heat. However, the rustic charm of wood burning stoves masks the fact that such fires produce some of the carcinogens found in cigarette smoking. Not only do such carcinogens threaten the people in the home, but wood burning stoves also pollute the air of the community. In cities like Portland, Oregon; Missoula, Montana; and

Denver, Colorado, <u>over one half</u> of the particulates (minute solids) in the winter air come from wood burning stoves, not from autos or industrialized factories.

The Sexual Revolution

General changes in societal mores and standards of living have a linkage of complex consequences that negatively impinge on our well-being. One example can be that of the "sexual revolution" whereby increased sexual contact had dire results far beyond gonorrhea and syphilis—both treatable by drug therapy. New strains of syphilis, and intestinal disorders that are immune to modern drug therapy, have emerged because of frequent sexual contact. An increase in hepatitis has brought death to many and a chronic debility to hundreds of thousands. Certain strains of herpes evolved with similar consequences. The spread of Acquired Immune Deficiency Syndrome (AIDS) is a frightening example of how changes in sexual mores seriously affect life chances. Many infected persons do not report the disease, and many others are unaware that they harbor the virus. Currently, there is no cure for this deadly disease. Without a change in our sexual mores and practices, and the adoption nationwide of effective prevention and control strategies, there is little chance of halting the spread of AIDS.

The downsides of the sexual revolution, in addition to those already mentioned, especially as they affect the young, remind us of the risks involved. For example, data from a variety sources reveal that sexually active girls are about three times more likely than their nonsexually active counterparts to become depressed and attempt suicide. "Hooking up" does not always have positive outcomes.

The Other Side of Affluence

With an increase in affluence comes the ability to indulge in consumption that eventually diminish life chances. Foods rich in saturated fats lead to both obesity and arteriosclerotic heart disease. Ironically, the cures for obesity can be pathological in themselves. *Aspartame*, the allegedly safe artificial sweetener, periodically is subjected to calls for its removal from public use. Saccharin has long been suspect for its link to cancer. Diet pills containing *phenylpropanolamine* (PPA) have been investigated as a link to kidney failure. Also, anorexia provides the deadly proof that concern about one's weight can be excessively and unconsciously carried to the antithesis of survival.

Nutritional Confusion

Nutritional behavior provides ample illustrations of how personal attitudes affect our well-being. The relationship between nutrition and health is a complex one. Experts differ on the effects of nutrition and there is considerable controversy as to the extent to which one can extrapolate results from animal studies to conclusions about humans. The national debate over the so-called "diet wars" has been characterized by one report as "turning the nation into a nutritional battlefield," where one finds "doctors, consumers, politicians and food marketers are all vying for control of the diet."[285] One side of this debate are the conservatives, who maintain that the average American diet supplies most of the nutrients people need. On the other side are the activists, who seek major changes in our eating habits. These clashing viewpoints led one biochemist to take note of "a too broad assumption that foods are either medicines or poisons." and that perhaps "the most important nutritional disease in America is *nutritional hypochondria.*"[286] In addition, physicians are recognizing that a person's genetic make-up plays a role in determining proper diets, and that quite literally, "One man's meat is another man's poison." The result of all this is a very perplexed public, yet one that is still tempted to accept the latest nutritional bulletin headlined through the mass media.

Despite the controversy and the confusion, there is a wide spectrum of government agencies, committees, and institutes who support the need for a balanced nutritional intake from the four main food groups, as well as a diet that limits fat contents to one third of the calories necessary for a particular weight group. The evidence is sufficiently convincing that one's food intake greatly affects the onset of a host of pathologies, such as myocardial degeneration, cardiovascular disease, and others.

Fats and Cholesterol. Limiting the intake of fats and cholesterol has emerged as one of the key factors in achieving a healthy body. High cholesterol levels have been linked to heart diseases by numerous investigators. Proper nutritional habits can keep such levels under control, particularly the dangerous low-density-lipoprotein (LDL) type. People who are overweight can lower their cholesterol level considerably by reducing. Certain fiber foods, such as carrots, apples, oats and soybeans, also help keep levels down. Aerobic exercise can produce a decrease in the percentage of LDL cholesterol in the blood.

The Significance of Lifestyle. For decades now the mortality rate from coronary heart disease has been steadily declining. This downward trend has coincided with impressive medical advances, on the one hand, *and* changes in diet and lifestyle, on the other. The question therefore arises as to which of these improvements has been most crucial. To find out, researchers compared the impact of a wide range of factors related to coronary-disease mortality. They found that five medical interventions saved a substantial number of lives: coronary-care units, drug therapy, treatment of high blood pressure, improved resuscitation techniques, and coronary by-pass surgery combined accounted for about 40 percent of the decline in mortality. However, two simple lifestyle changes—reduction of fat consumption and cigarette smoking—had even more impact. Together, they accounted for over half of the decline.

Obesity: A Major Culprit.

Being overweight has reached epidemic proportions in the United States and Canada.[287] Excessive weight is increasingly identified as the culprit behind many conditions of heart disease, hypertension, diabetes, and certain cancers. It is a major factor in premature death. Studies show, for example, that regardless of smoking habits, obese men have higher death rates from cancer of the colon, rectum and prostate, while overweight females have higher mortality rates from cancers of the gallbladder, cervix, uterus, ovaries and breast. There is general agreement that a reduction in food-intake, eating a variety of foods in moderation, and maintaining a normal weight would go a long ways towards averting the potential threats to life posed by obesity. As anyone who has tried to adhere to this common sense approach knows, it is easier said than done.

Americans engaged in the constant "battle of the bulge" implicitly recognize the dangers to their personal well-being that can be provoked by excessive pounds. While estimates vary, it appears that at least half of adult women and a fourth of adult men in the United States are dieting at any one time. Each year millions swarm to thousands of centers offering commercial weight-reduction programs and their associated diets. They sometimes spend considerable sums of money to achieve the promise of a slimmer body offered by these programs. Most succeed in temporarily losing weight, at which point they often terminate the program. To their chagrin, however, the vast majority regain that weight within weeks or months.[288] Unable to maintain their compliance regimen, and keep the pounds off, they then return to the program to slim down once again. Repeated cycles of this kind are quite common. (The problem is exacerbated by the natural tendency to gain weight with age). Many scientists caution that this "yo-yo" pattern of weight change can be life-threatening.[289] A long-term survey of residents of Framingham, Massachusetts revealed that people whose weight rose and fell repeatedly over many years had a significantly higher incidence of heart disease and premature death than people whose weight remained stable.[290] The reasons for this effect are unclear. One theory why this pattern of weight changes is hazardous suggests that pounds lost from the lower part of the body may be gained back in the upper part. Excess fat above the waistline has been linked with a higher risk of heart disease. *Permanent* weight loss is a goal that extends beyond the tempting promises of commercial diet programs. The Framingham experience reaffirms the well-established principle that safe weight-loss can best be achieved by adopting lifelong, prudent eating habits along with regular exercise.

The Economy and Human Casualties

Just as affluence affects our lifestyle, which in turns influences our chances of staying alive, so do fluctuations in the economic structure of our nation. Researchers have found that a certain increase in the unemployment rate is followed by a concomitant rise in the overall mortality rate. More specifically, they discovered that changes in the unemployment rate and other economic measures are strongly correlated with various indicators of medical or social pathology. These include mortality from cardiovascular and renal disease, the rate of first admissions to mental hospitals, the suicide rate, the rate of reported crime, and the homicide rate.[291] Moreover, it appears that these effects continue for a considerable period (as long as 15 years later in some instances) after the initial economic shock.

The adverse health consequences resulting from economic fluctuations are concentrated among the lower-income and minority groups in the society. Even during normal economic circumstances, members of these groups suffer from a combination of stress, poor diet, and inadequate medical care. However, radical changes in the economy often widen the disparity between the living conditions of the upper and lower classes, especially the poor. It is not surprising, therefore, that rising rates of several of the most severe pathologies correlate with an increase in social inequality.[292] In other words, the life chances of the poor are much more sensitive to major shifts in the economy or to government policies which affect their economic well-being. The above research found, for example, that government-mandated decreases in Aid for Dependent Children payments were associated with an immediate rise in the infant mortality rate. Whether a similar outcome will result from then more recent mandated welfare reform remains to be seen.

Longitudinal data on a variety of countries reveal a persistent inverse relationship between parental social class and infant mortality. Such findings confirm the "classic rule," that unfavorable social conditions increases the probability of early death. In other words, mortality tends to be lowest in the highest social class and then progressively increases with decreases in social class.[293] This rule also prevails at the international level where cross-nation comparisons reveal wide disparities in infant and maternal mortality. In modern or developed nations children under five account for only a small proportion of all deaths each year. But their counterparts in developing countries account for up to 80 percent of all deaths each year. Similarly, whereas in most developed countries maternal deaths account for less than two percent of all deaths among women of child-bearing age, the figure is significantly higher in many regions of undeveloped nations. Moreover, many other women in the latter countries suffer from illnesses related to pregnancy, abortion, or childbirth.[294]

The social inequality of death and survivorship has long been noted by social analysts. This classic rule has little chance of being altered until the society finds the will and the means to extend the benefits of good health to our most vulnerable populations. However, this societal effort, to be most effective, must also be accompanied by a degree of personal responsibility. It has been argued that medical care, by itself, will not eliminate or even reduce to minimal levels the devastating impact of any of the various health problems that are borne by the poor—whether one is talking about the devastating impact of chronic disease on the disadvantaged, or the rate of infant mortality, or the burden of homicide and violence. In order to extend the benefits of good health to everyone it will be necessary to create among the most vulnerable populations a "culture of character," that is, "a culture, or a way of thinking and being, that actively promotes responsible behavior and the adoption of lifestyles that are maximally conducive to good health."[295] This represents prevention in the broadest sense, and is an absolute necessity for achieving good health.

Infant Mortality: A Case In Point

Some support for this perspective comes from an analysis of infant mortality. It turns out that, like most propositions involving human behavior, the previously mentioned classic rule is much more complex then we have thus far indicated, and may miss the mark in terms of its implications for correcting the problem. Despite a variety of initiatives and programs implemented over the past several decades, the proportion of babies in the United States dying before their first birthday, while showing some decline, is still higher than that of most industrialized countries. Slow progress in this area has led some to question the presumption that lowering material poverty and providing adequate health care will solve the problem of infant survival.

In this connection Eberstadt, notes that economic data are unable to explain why some poorer groups in this country have lower infant-mortality rates than some richer groups.[296] Asians and Pacific Islanders, for example, have a higher poverty rate than whites in America, yet their infant mortality rate is lower. Again, infant death rates for Hispanic Americans and non-Hispanic whites are about equal, despite the fact that the poverty rate for Hispanic children is more than twice as high. Comparisons between blacks and Puerto Rico residents raise similar questions about the role of economics. Blacks on any number of measures are the more affluent of the two; yet their infant mortality rate is significantly higher.

Inadequate medical care also fails to provide a fully satisfactory explanation of lower infant survival rates. It has been consistently shown, for example, that the lower a baby's birth weight the greater the risk of premature death. Infant mortality rates are roughly 20 times higher for low-birth weight babies than for those above 5.5 pounds at delivery. Yet the chances of an infant surviving at any given high-risk birth weight were substantially better in the United States than in Norway or Japan—two countries with the lowest infant mortality rate. The American advantage here, which held for both blacks and whites, suggests that this country's infant health services are generally good and broadly available.

It appears then that our infant mortality problem may have less to do with the survival chances of any low birth weight baby than with the unusually large numbers of infants born into high-risk categories. Among blacks, the incidence of low birth weight is not only higher than that of virtually any other Western population, but also twice as high as whites in the United States. Yet the incidence among U.S. whites is also high—nearly twice that of Norway, for instance. Why does this country produce so many low-birth weight babies? For Eberstadt a large part of the answer can be attributed to a lack of parental responsibility. "The evidence suggests that the attitudes, practices and lifestyles of many American parents—including many who are neither poor nor poorly educated—are exposing U.S. babies to unfamiliar and unnecessary hazards." That evidence includes the following:

1. A survey of mothers by the Center for Disease Control (CDC) found that poorer white women had the same incidence of low birth weight as more affluent mothers. However, those babies described as "unwanted or mistimed" experi-

enced much greater risks of low birth weight than those portrayed as "wanted at conception."

2. CDC data also show that irrespective of the mother's age or race, babies born out-of-wedlock are most likely to exhibit low birth weight and higher infant mortality. The argument that these correlations reflect the social disadvantages characteristic of unwed mothers is difficult to sustain because, "illegitimacy has been going mainstream." He notes that over half of all babies born out-of-wedlock each year are to white mothers, and that more are to mothers 25 years or older, than to teenagers. More than a fourth of the white, single mothers in their early 30's now have at least some college education.

3. Another CDC study revealed that infant mortality rates were higher for unmarried mothers who were college graduates than for married grade-school dropouts. This held true for both blacks and whites. How does one explain this? Again, risky behavior on the part of parents-to-be may play a large role. A Missouri study of 60,000 births showed a strong inverse relationship between a mother's years of education and her propensity to smoke during pregnancy. Nevertheless, unwed college graduates, regardless of race, were more apt to smoke during pregnancy than the average married woman—even though the latter had almost an even chance of being a high school drop-out.

4. Illegal drug use during pregnancy can also hurt a fetus. It is widely presumed that such behavior is characteristic mainly of impoverished, inner city, minority populations. However, research conducted in Rhode Island suggests a different story. The state Department of Health tested a sample of women-in labor for illicit drugs. About 7 1/2 percent tested positive for one or more illicit drugs. Those who were black, young, or poor were more likely to test positive. Surprisingly, however, fully 7% of the white mothers also tested positive, and women 25 years or older showed a similar rate. Moreover, nearly 7 percent of those not classified as being in poverty tested positive.

All of this leads Eberstadt to conclude that unless such dangerous parental behavior is somehow corrected, infant survival will remain unnecessarily problematic. He echoes the admonition of the Secretary of Health with respect to individual responsibility when he states that despite the continued progress made in reducing the infant mortality rate—through medical advances and increased health expenditures—that rate is likely to remain needlessly high unless the problem of hazardous parental behavior is somehow controlled. Many have argued that governmental policy should be framed so as not only to promote longevity, but also to ensure greater adherence to model parental behavior as well. Indeed, many programs designed to improve the nation's health often require parental cooperation, and therefore are, by implication, also aimed at strengthening the family unit. In the final analysis, however, infant survival is dependent on a variety of influences—advances in medical technology, parental cooperation, **and** access to pre-natal care.

The lower class finds it particularly difficult to obtain proper medical care. A survey of the hospital care provided to babies in California found that newborn infants without health insurance received significantly fewer medical services than newborns covered by health insurance. There was a strong suggestion that physicians and hospitals consciously or unconsciously discriminate against patients whose ability to pay for care is limited. They conclude that "fewer hospital services to vulnerable groups likely to be at higher risk during the first days of life" indicate evidence of serious inequity.[297]

Preventive care is, in fact, essential to insure that more babies are born healthy and stay healthy. Otherwise we are left with a reliance on modern technology to save very sick babies. That alone, however, will not solve the problem. On the other hand, limitations on access to care can certainly exacerbate it and pose serious threats to survival.

This inequity in health care is, of course, by no means confined to infants. At the present time more than 45 million Americans have no health insurance. This figure is likely to increase as more employers now drop coverage or offer plans that are too expensive for many people. Without such coverage they become particularly vulnerable to extended periods of poor health and life-threatening illnesses. There is good evidence, for example, that uninsured and Medicaid covered patients have more health problems and fare less well after receiving medical care than those with access to private insurance. A study of inpatient records by a research team at the Center for Health Policy Studies at Georgetown University revealed that death rates for uninsured hospital patients were as much as triple the rates for those with insurance.[298] Another team examined hospital discharge data for Massachusetts and found that uninsured persons who were hospitalized for a heart attack faced a much higher risk of dying than their insured counterparts, despite the availability of an uncompensated care pool for paying hospitals to treat the uninsured. Moreover, the uninsured patients were less likely than the insured to undergo cardiac procedures, such as angioplasty and coronary artery bypass surgery. The uninsureds' higher death rate and lower procedures rate suggest that they received differential treatment compared with those insured.[299]

The conditions of social inequality, whether in general or in more specific contexts, such as the health care system, continues to reduce the life chances of millions of people in the wealthiest industrialized nation in the world. An analysis of mortality data for Medicare patients in nearly 6,000 hospitals is illustrative.[300] It revealed that over 100 of them, may in our large cities and the rural South, had significantly higher death rates for elderly patients than would be expected, given the patients ages and medical histories. Administrators at a number of these contended that the methodology and the data for the study were seriously flawed, and did not take into account the demography of the population served by a particular institution, for example, their socio-economic status. It is true that many of the hospitals with consistently higher-than-expected death rates served some of the poorest urban populations in the United States and its territories. Few of the administrators, however, would question that regional and demographic conditions are closely linked to the quality of the health care system and its influence on a patient's ability to survive.

Summary

This chapter has emphasized the need to view life chances in the broad context of American society. Patterns of mortality are not randomly distributed. They reflect an array of factors that underscore the close link between societal conditions and their impact on the individual. Technological and social changes can be profound in promoting or threatening the ability to stay alive. Our discussion leads to the conclusion that there is still a great need to develop and implement a societal commitment to longevity and to improving the quality of life. Such a commitment would be a significant impetus in achieving the overall goal that the government has established for reducing the risks of premature death.

11

Ecological Threats to Survival

Environmental Pollution

Throughout most of history humans have depended on the natural ecosystems of the earth in order to survive. However, over time the agricultural and industrial revolutions gave them greater control over the extent and dimensions of that dependency. They could, for example, grow their own food or create new sources of energy. Much beneficial progress in the human condition can be attributed to man's progressive ability to manipulate nature. However, with that progress also came the ability to damage the environment and threaten the fragile ecological, sociological, and economic compatibility essential to life support systems on earth.

> Industrial societies have evolved under the influence of a political-economic reward system and a technological revolution that literally views the environment as infinite in its waste absorbing capabilities, if not in resource producing capability as well. As such they are not ecologically feasible in the long term. It is precisely their inconsistencies with the laws of material and energy balance under the pressures of an expanding human population that are generating the environmental crisis.[301]

It was the growing recognition of that crisis that brought representatives of the world's governments together in Rio De Janeiro, Brazil, in June, 1992, to the first so-called Earth Summit, or more precisely, the United Nations Conference on Environment and Development. Their discussions were aimed at developing equitable resolutions to a difficult and fundamental dilemma, namely, "how to pursue economic growth and combat poverty while at the same time protecting the interacting web of atmosphere, water, soil and biological organisms on which human life depends."[302] This complex task will not be easy.

Threats to the Biosphere. Among the formidable worldwide problems facing the Summit participants were: 1) Bad Air. Every day billions of people inhale smog, sulfur dioxide, acid rain, carbon monoxide and other toxic pollutants; 2) Dirty Water. Sewage, soil erosion, pesticides and toxic waste have defiled drinking water and destroyed coastal habitats; 3) Loss of forests. The destruction of trees is resulting in erosion, flooding, desertification, and global warming; 4) Soil Degradation. Over one-tenth of the earth's soil has already been degraded by chemicals, erosion, and overuse; 5) Ozone Depletion. Unless halted, the stratospheric ozone shield which protects the earth from excessive and biologically harmful ultraviolet light might be depleted by 10 percent by the end of this century in the temperate zones. Predictions include drought, change in agricultural patterns, and a rise in skin cancer rates; (6) Global Warming. Buildup of gases is causing the planet to heat up—the so-called greenhouse effect. Eight of the ten warmest years on record have occurred in recent decades. Earth's temperature may increase several degrees over the next century; 7) Overpopulation. Global population, which stood at 2.5 billion only 55 years ago, is now over 6 billion, and might increase to 10 billion by the middle of the next century. There is considerable concern over the ability of nature to sustain this proliferation of people; 8) Endangered Species. One-fourth of the earth's current species of plants and animals may be extinct within the next two or three decades. In some countries many of the necessary habitats for their survival have already been destroyed by human encroachment.

Achieving worldwide consensus and cooperation on strategies for resolving the growing deterioration of the biosphere will be extremely difficult, and costly. It is compounded by the fact that much scientific uncertainty and disagreement surround the various dimensions of the problem, and the degree to which the biosphere is, in fact, in jeopardy. Polemics and rhetoric abound over the issues, with considerable confusion as the result. Charges and countercharges attacking the motivations of advocates on either side of this debate appear regularly in the lay and scientific literature.[303] It is difficult for the public to decipher the mass of contradictory evidence offered by the scientific, economic, and political proponents of strategies proposed to deal with environmental issues. There is, nevertheless, a growing awareness that community and corporate endeavors related to advancing technology pose ecological threats at the societal level which often severely constrain the spectrum of individual choices related to life preservation.

This is especially apparent with respect to the effects of environmental contamination on human health. Some pollutants have been accumulating at increased rates since mid-twentieth century. Among these are rising air pollution, pesticide residues that infiltrate the soil and adulterate the food chains, wide-spread penetration of organic and mineral wastes and other contaminants in our rivers, lakes, and oceans, and fallout of isotopes with long half-lives. These and other alterations of the environment, which have resulted from large-scale social and economic changes, can induce old and new forms of disabilities and reduce the life expectancy of countless individuals.[304]

In this chapter we want to examine environmental hazards as they impact our health and welfare—but in a very select fashion. The literature on this topic has mushroomed to the point where no single analysis can ever hope to but scratch the surface. Moreover, the list of presumed risks to our health and longevity continues to lengthen at a pace which quickly overwhelms one's psychological capacity to deal with it. The range of those risks embraces deadly pollutants that we may be breathing in our homes or at work (the "sick-building syndrome") to the poisonous fumes escaping from the local crematorium. Descriptions such as the one below make you want to flee outside to breathe fresh air:

> The home, after all, is a place where oil, gas, wood and tobacco are burned (giving off nitrogen dioxide, carbon monoxide and hydrocarbons); it offers a collection of microclimates ideal for the cultivation of microorganisms (including fungi, nematodes and the bacteria that cause Legionnaire's disease among other ailments); it is a place where countless chemical products invisibly exude their volatile components, including styrene from plastics and benzene from solvents. Manufactured-wood products, such as particleboard and plywood, give off poisonous formaldehyde, and even the very soil beneath the foundation can emit radioactive radon gas.[305]

The problem is that we know relatively little about how serious a threat many of the pollutants in the air of our homes are to our health. The dangers of some, like radon or asbestos fibers, are clear and should be of concern. For many indoor pollutants, however, the jury is still out. Chemical toxins in the home pose similar problems. The Environmental Protection Agency has reported that the various toxins found in our homes are three times more likely to cause cancer than the outside airborne pollutants, even in areas next to chemical plants. Researchers, however, face considerable difficulty in developing concrete evidence that the mere presence of toxins in the average home has *directly* caused the demise of one or more of its occupants.

Nevertheless, the link between air pollution (indoor or outdoor) and our health and longevity is a legitimate and growing area of concern. Homes and work places often do contain dangerous chemicals. Indeed, it's been estimated that more than 50,000 chemical compounds can be found in an average household.[306] Many of these are potential hazards. But establishing their actual impact on our well-being is neither simple nor easy.[307] In the following pages we shift the focus to outside the home, concentrating on those involuntary risks that people incur from some of the major external pollutants.

Contaminated Communities

Of particular concern are the potential calamities posed by industrial chemical hazards, which often have long-term health consequences. In the United States alone, it has been estimated that every day the chemical and petroleum industries produce about 275 million gallons of gasoline, 2.5 million pounds of pesticides and herbicides, and nearly 723,000 tons of dangerous wastes."[308] Also, each day about a quarter million loads of hazardous materials, mostly petrochemicals, are transported across the nation by railroad or over our roads. While fatal accidents have been few, the possibility of their occurrence is of constant concern and worry, to both the manufacturers and the public alike. Moreover, the toxic residue from these petrochemicals can have dramatic outcomes. For example, the residents of Times Beach, Missouri were forced to abandon permanently their town when it was discovered that the water and ground were contaminated with dangerous levels of *dioxin*, a highly potent poison capable of producing cancer, genetic damage, and a variety of other serious health problems. The community, with its boarded up windows and empty streets, now resembles a ghost town. Its former residents remain apprehensive over the possible long-term health consequences of having lived in that contaminated environment.

Several other communities have been struck by toxic pollution, leaving in its wake the destruction of neighborhoods, emotional as well as financial trauma, illness and long-term health effects and, in many instances, eventual death. The population of toxic victims is growing in the United States and elsewhere in the world. One analysis of these contaminated communities has characterized widespread toxic exposure as a new "technological plague," causing physical, psychological, social, and cultural effects among hundreds of residential communities.[309] A subtle but important consequence of such exposure is the disruption of our *lifescape*, a term that refers to both our idiosyncratic and shared paradigms for understanding the world. People seldom become aware of their lifescapes until some condition or event—like the threats of toxic exposure—disrupts their lifestyle or somehow disconfirms their operating assumptions about the worlds in which they live. Moreover:

...disconfirmation of the lifescape may challenge core assumptions of the overall society. For example, toxic exposure directly assails several fundamental social beliefs: that humans have dominion over nature; that personal control over one's destiny is possible; that technology and science are forces of progress only; that risks necessary for the good life are acceptable; that people get what they deserve; that experts know best; that the marketplace is self-regulating; that one's home is one's castle; that people have the right to do what they wish on their own property; and that government exists to help (pp. 11-12).

Most of us would find it difficult to discard such beliefs. But that possibility arises with each encounter with toxic exposure and the stressful process of coping with its immediate and long-term damaging effects. Too often such encounters lead to a distrust of those assigned the tasks of resolving the crisis and rescuing the victims from their plight. Government agencies and their minions (scientists, engineers, etc.), in particular, are often viewed as biased toward industry. The result is conflict instead of collaboration between government and the exposed citizens. Disappointed in the bureaucratic response, individuals increasingly find themselves forced to organize at the grass roots level in order to achieve a satisfactory solution to the problem. We shall have more to say later about the process of citizen initiative as a strategy in getting their concerns adequately represented in resolving life-threatening conditions brought on by environmental pollution.

Primary and Secondary Disasters

Industrial hazards can be roughly divided into primary and secondary disasters.[310] Primary disasters are those which strike quickly and without warning and kill instantly and widely. The Bhopal tragedy, in which deadly gas escaped from a plant in India and killed many people, would be classified as a primary disaster. Fortunately, such large-scale man-made tragedies are extremely rare, especially in the more developed countries.[311] Increased public concern over the potential threats to survival posed by the voluminous production and transportation of hazardous materials, coupled with growing and elaborate governmental regulations, has motivated the chemical companies to achieve greater safety systems in the design and operation of their facilities. While the safety record has significantly improved, violent chemical explosions, fires, or lethal gas leaks can, and do, periodically occur. The explosion of a series of gas tanks in San Juan Ixhuatepec, a suburb of Mexico City, which killed over 450 people, and the widespread destruction of underground sewers in Guatemala, which took so many innocent victims, are tragic reminders of the need to monitor constantly these industrial systems. The oil and gas industries are illustrative here. The United States has over 200 operating oil refineries, more than a quarter of a million oil pipelines, and more than a million miles of natural gas conduits.

> Sometimes refineries and storage tanks are clumped together like rusting armadas of iron behemoths, belching smoke into the sky. Along the New Jersey Turnpike, near the towns of Linden and Carteret many oil storage tanks are higher than a ten-story apartment building. Should a plane from nearby Newark International Airport crash into that complex, the resulting fireball could engulf one of the most heavily populated areas of the nation.[312]

Little wonder that fire drills at the plants in this area have been substantially increased!

Disposal of wastes from so-called "hi-tech" industries can also lead to secondary disasters, those that result in the slow poisoning of the soil and water. The dumping of toxic chemical and radioactive wastes into rivers and oceans, or on or under the ground, are prime examples of this category. The long-term health repercussions of such practices, and the threat they pose to the ecology and human survival, have received widespread publicity in the mass media and in both the lay and scientific communities. The ecological stress caused by the spreading contamination of our coastal waters by millions of tons of discharged sewage, garbage, toxic chemicals and other contaminants is increasingly recognized as a national crisis.

Again, the energy industry is a good example. In many areas of America, but especially west of the Mississippi, there are thousands of oil and gas wells that were abandoned at the end of their productive life. The Environmental Protection Agency estimates that there are more than a million of these abandoned wells and that about 200,000 or more of them may not be properly plugged. Many of these problem wells date back to an earlier period before the industry was regulated or adequate records were kept. The *New York Times* article which called attention to this matter quotes a director of a county health department in West Texas as saying: "We've found leaking wells from the old days that were rock-plugged, bucket-plugged, tree-stump-plugged and even one plugged with nothing more than a glass jug because back then they just stuck whatever they had down the hole." Sometimes they are simply capped with a metal plate and covered with dirt. Because they often are unable to prevent seepage, an untold number have become conduits for noxious liquids comprised of a brine that can be four times saltier than sea water and laced with radioactivity, heavy metals and other toxins. Over time these fluids slowly and insidiously percolate upward from deep below the earth's surface to destroy eventually crops and contaminate drinking water.[313]

The dangers posed by oil field contamination have only recently attracted the attention of state government and industry officials. Unfortunately, the monies needed to fix the problem, either by imposing new taxes or fees on companies drilling or operating oil wells, are hard to come by. Moreover, when low prices and exhausted fields drive down production, the result often is a rise in bankrupt operators who then abandon more wells. The practice of forcefully injecting vast quantities of brine back into a depleted well, in order to dispose of it or to increase pressure in the oil-bearing formation so that more crude can be extracted from a nearby active well, further compounds the danger. It can threaten essential fresh water aquifers, lead to extensive and critical environmental damage, and place both human beings and wildlife at risk. The health of these aquifers is of particular concern in places where they feed large river systems—systems upon which major cities, ranches, farms, and electric power plants are so dependent.

Clearly, secondary disasters can have long-term and widespread reverberation, not only for those who live near oil fields, or in America, but everywhere. The world is being impacted by an ever-growing accumulation of various poisonous wastes as well as radioactive sludge.[314] It is generally agreed that the vast majority of all the toxic chemicals produced is not disposed of properly. Until recently, it was commonplace practice simply to dump dangerous amounts wherever, with little regard for environmental damage, and where they could gradually permeate the ground and eventually enter water supplies. One of the most widely publicized instances of this is the Love Canal in Niagara Falls. For two decades the Hooker Chemical Company dumped millions of barrels of industrial wastes into a nearby landfill. Eventually, the land was covered over and sold to the city. Subsequently, single family homes residences were erected there.

Later the basements of many of the homes were infiltrated with toxic wastes seeping through the walls and foundations. Families began to experience unusual levels of asthma, kidney disease, hepatitis, and birth defects. Physical, psychological, and social distress were much in evidence. Dozens of families had to be evacuated from the site, and some of their houses were purchased from them by the state. Eventually the area was largely abandoned, and "the words "Love Canal" became synonymous with poison."[315]

Environmental Damage versus Economic Welfare. The Environmental Protection Agency has been charged with the major responsibility of identifying and overseeing the clean-up of the thousands of hazardous waste sites which now exist across the nation. Unfortunately, its efforts have too often been compromised by bureaucratic red-tape and mismanagement, as well as by political intrusions. The monumental effort and resources required to rectify the widespread environmental damage can easily discourage even those most staunchly committed to the task. Many in the public sector understandably often resist such efforts if they are viewed as threats to their economic welfare, for example, by requiring a local plant to shut down or relocate, thereby leaving people without jobs. Still others have, over time, developed a fatalistic attitude toward the potential hazards of nearby industry. "There isn't much I can do about it." Or, "It's the only game in town." Thus, they rationalize that the job security provided by this or that industry is worth the risk.

Achieving a sensible balance between activities which serve the economic interests of industry and community, with actions aimed at minimizing dangerous threats to the environment, is admittedly a complex and difficult task. Some believe it is an impossible task. But a constant striving to achieve that objective everywhere is essential if people and planet are to survive. It will require an *ethical imperative* which soundly rejects the "profit at all costs" mentality which in the long-run is self-destructive. That imperative must also hold business, industry, and government accountable whenever their actions pose unacceptable risks to people and the environment. To compromise the rational balance between economic benefits and ecological risks is to invite eventual disaster, disease, and death.[316]

Pesticides: The Ubiquitous Dilemma

More than fifty years ago Rachel Carson published her best-selling and controversial book *Silent Spring,* which exposed the devastation wrought by agricultural pesticides.[317] These chemical compounds, so essential to food production, are also poisonous. A minute proportion, perhaps less than 1 percent, actually reaches the pests it is intended to control or eradicate. The remainder ends up as contaminants in water, residues on produce, and noxious fallout on farm field hands. Its been estimated that worldwide pesticides each year fatally poison 10,000 people, injure hundreds of thousands more, and leave millions of others vulnerable to increased cancer, reproductive problems, and birth defects resulting from low-level, chronic exposure. These compounds pose a major life and death dilemma. We are dependent on them for maintaining adequate levels of agricultural products; yet they pose a threat to human health and welfare. Their widespread use can pose hard choices. "We can't seem to do without pesticides; but can we live with their consequences?"[318]

Many of these were approved for use years ago when the science of toxology was still in its infancy and lab tests were rudimentary. In some instances, fraudulent data apparently were used to gain approval. Under current law, the EPA is required to reevaluate *all* pesticides now being used. The catch in that legislation is that the EPA does not have to institute a ban on any pesticide unless the risk it carries outweighs its economic benefit.[319] As one might guess, relatively few bans have been issued. In a ten year period, only 5 pesticides were banned and 23 others restricted because of their potential hazard. Even in these cases, however, the compounds may continue to linger in the environment for many years after. DDT is a well-known example of this lingering effect. Although its use has been banned in the United States since 1972, it can be stored in the body's fatty tissues for decades. In 1993 researchers established a statistical link between exposure to this pesticide and the risk of breast cancer.[320] The sample of subjects was small, and comprised primarily of Caucasian New York women from upper socioeconomic backgrounds. The findings suggest that the pesticide may be one of the factors underlying the sharp rise in the incidence of breast cancer among women over 50 years age. They are among the generation which had the greatest exposure to the pesticide before it was banned.

A significant number of pesticides banned in the United States subsequently find their way back via crops imported from Third World countries. In addition, tests have detected amounts of pesticide residue in some samples of fruits and vegetables grown here, which greatly exceed the prescribed limits. Increasing amounts of these chemicals are also finding their way into ground water, especially in agricultural states.

Surprisingly, despite the widespread use of modern pesticides and its accompanying technology, today we evidently lose about the same percentage of the nation's crops to insects as we did fifty years ago! This is largely due to an unanticipated consequence, namely, the chemicals used often annihilate the natural predators of the targeted insects. The insects then become increasingly resistant to subsequent applications of the pesticide. The problems of pesticide resistance and pesticide hazards strongly suggest a need both for reforming their use, for example, by employing new herbicides less hazardous to the environment, and for reducing their overall deployment through improved pest management programs.[321]

Another unanticipated consequence results from the complex interactions between pesticides and prescription drugs. Such interactions are increasingly apt to occur given the growth in everyday chemical products, such as lawn-care pesticide products, used around the home, and the use of prescribed drugs. Exposure to combinations of toxic chemicals and drugs are suspected of causing serious health problems, and can be fatal. In one recent case, a man was poisoned by an organophosphate pesticide (***diazinon***) used to treat the yard and lawn. An investigation strongly suggested that the poison was absorbed through his skin and by inhaling the pesticide fumes. The body normally flushes away small or moderate amounts of this compound. However, in this case the situation was complicated by the fact that the man was taking prescribed daily doses of ***Tagamet***, a widely used ulcer drug. Medical scientists believe that this medication suppressed the normal function of the liver in metabolizing the pesticide and expelling it. Consequently, it accumulated in his body and hence became more potent in its assault on the nervous system. Subsequently he developed testicular cancer and a host of other serious health problems.[322] Both the makers of the pesticide and the drug denied their products were in any way responsible, arguing that they are safe when used correctly. A lawsuit filed against the two companies was unsuccessful.

No government agency conducts routine tests for these kinds of interactions. Manufacturers are not required to perform tests for interactions between their products and prescription drugs. It may be an impossible task, given the thousands of such products now on the market, and given the fact that drug metabolism varies widely by age, physique, sex, ethnic group, and other factors. The proportion of our population being exposed each year to toxic pesticides has steadily increased, with an associated rise in people requiring treatment in health-care facilities. There have been instances of accidental exposure which has resulted in death. But these acute exposures are only part of the problem. Of equal if not greater concern is the fact that many people may be vulnerable to chronic, low-level exposure to pesticides that can produce severe health problems over time. Accumulation of these toxins in the body tissue heightens the risk for cancer, birth defects and damage to the liver, kidneys, and the nervous system. There apparently is little public awareness of these risks. "Many do-it-yourselfers still don't read the labels. Many who do read them can't understand what they say, and others don't understand the dangers of failing to follow the instructions."[323] Even following the instructions may not preclude eventual ill effects. At present, many of the interaction mechanisms between pesticides and drugs are little understood.

Scientists disagree over the relative threat, to humans and the environment, of pesticides. Some argue that the small amounts to which we are actually exposed are harmless. Others contend that *any* amount is unacceptable, since many of the currently used fungicides are known to be detrimental to human health. Still others take the position that the thousands of natural carcinogens found in foods pose risks vastly greater than the comparatively small hazards of man-made synthetic pesticides. The most recent evidence indicates that there are large and small risks within both categories. In the face of uncertainties concerning the use of pesticides, regulatory agencies typically favor rules that minimize the assumption of unnecessary risk on the part of the public. *Consumer Reports*, which conducted an intensive analysis of the issues surrounding this matter, concluded that in the final analysis: "The debate over regulating pesticides in foods is inherently a political one, a battle over how society should manage risks and allocate limited cancer-prevention resources."[324] Given the uncertainties, and the ongoing battle between the proponents and opponents of pesticide use, prudence would dictate the exercise of considerable caution in the handling of and exposure to such products. As we have seen, one's life may depend on it.

Avoiding the Engineering Fallacy

If challenges to the environmental threats we face ultimately are to succeed, we will have to give up what Edelstein has termed *the engineering fallacy*. This fallacy assumes that problems can be isolated and resolved without having to take into account the complicated and uncertain societal contexts in which they occur. As a result, we have often erroneously assumed that problems have been solved:

> only to realize later that they have reemerged, demanding new solutions. In this way, the era of indiscriminate dumping gave way to landfilling, or discriminate dumping. When landfilling subsequently came to be recognized as an abject failure, dumping gave way to incineration and deep-well injection. With each shift, society is convinced that it has "solved" the problems of hazardous waste.[325]

In other words, society has assumed a patch-it-up mode, one that places tremendous energy and resources on treating symptoms (for example, air pollution) rather than challenging the underlying attitudes, values, and their related lifestyles (for example, the emphasis on personal automobiles over public transportation) that allow the problem to develop in the first place.

An unquestioning faith in engineered solutions to various threats fails to comprehend that environmental problems reflect more basic issues having to do with some of our fundamental values. Edelstein puts this in the form of a *meta-issue*, asking, "Why have we come to accept contamination as a necessary cost of the good life? Said another way—why have we come to accept the polluting life as good?" One can think of any number of similar questions. For example, "Why have we come to view disposable containers as acceptable?" (Remember when the milkman collected the empty bottles outside our door so that they could be cleaned and reused?) Until we are willing to address important meta-issues, those which reflect our philosophy of living, environmental contamination will continue to pose serious threats to the human condition.

Natural Disasters

There are a host of natural disasters that always have the potential to terminate lives and for which there is often little forewarning and protection—hurricanes, tornados, tsunamis, earthquakes, to name just a few. Recent hurricane Katrina was so devastating that it literally wiped out the entire city of New Orleans, cost many lives, billions in physical damage and economic collapse. The disaster forced the population to scatter over several states and it will be years before their old neighborhoods are habitable. It appears that much of the population that left will not return. Obviously, the consequences of this disaster are national and international in scope. New Orleans will remain vulnerable despite its reconstructed levies because of its location. This raises the question, given the knowledge of the vulnerability of the location of New Orleans why anyone would deliberately choose to risk the harm of another natural disaster by settling there. The annual hurricane season poses very similar questions to all those who choose to live along the East coast. Apparently the inhabitant weigh the risk against the benefits and elect the risks.

12

The Health Care Providers

Survival and the Ethical Imperative

Americans spend billions of dollars on health care each year. Anywhere from a fourth to one-third or more of that cost has been attributed to overpriced, useless, and sometimes even harmful treatments, along with an inflated bureaucracy. That medical bureaucracy alone consumes about one-fifth of the total amount spent each year. The United States spends a greater percentage of its gross national product on health care than any other developed country in the world. Yet we are no healthier than the people in comparable developed countries that spend half what we do, and still provide health care for all their citizens.[326] Moreover, our health care system is undermined by wide scale waste and fraud amounting to tens of billions of dollars each year.[327] Few, if any, of those involved in the management of our health care system would disagree with this assessment.

Consumer Reports conservatively estimates that about twenty percent of the money we spend on health care is for procedures and services that are unnecessary. Included here would be needlessly high rates for such costly interventions as caesarean deliveries and hysterectomies, as well as many other procedures.[328] Such overtreatment has been documented by *outcome analyses*, which track medical cases to determine if and when specific procedures, for example, hysterectomies, justify their risks and drawbacks. Analysts involved with outcome analyses have concluded that: "Almost every study that has seriously looked for overuse has discovered it, and virtually every time at least double-digit overuse has been found."[329] Another twenty percent or more of the money spent on health care goes to days in the hospital that are unwarranted. We know that the number of days patients spend in the hospital can in fact be significantly lowered without adversely affecting their health. Costs of hospitalization account for almost 40 percent of national health care expenditures.

The combined dollar amount for overuse of medical services and administrative inefficiency is estimated to be at least $200 billion a year, and probably much more. However, this figure does not include the cost of other factors, such as escalating physicians' fees, and new diagnostic technologies, drugs, and procedures. Nor does it include the cost of various types of medical fraud—ordering unnecessary tests and procedures, billing for services never rendered, falsifying reimbursement codes to collect more than the usual payment for service, submitting inflated bills for supplies and medical devices, and various kickback schemes. The government estimates fraud could be absorbing up to 10 percent of the total health-care budget.

The high cost of our health care system might be justified if it resulted in making us healthier than people in other countries. But the evidence shows that it does not. A comparison of the health status of the people in the 24 industrialized nations reveals that the United States ranks 21st in infant mortality, 17th in male life expectancy, and 16th in female life expectancy. Another comparison with nine industrialized European nations with respect to the availability of high-quality primary care, various public-health indicators, and overall satisfaction with the value of health care, ranked this country at or near the bottom in all three areas.[330]

Escalating and excessive physician fees are a significant factor in the nation's spiraling health care costs. Physicians often require unnecessary procedures which have the effect of raising the price of their services. The *Reports* refers to this practice of creating a medical need by the people who profit from it as *the law of induced demand*, "and it's rampant" (p. 438). Utilization of the latest medical technologies is particularly profitable, especially those associated with cardiac catherization, angioplasty, bypass surgery, and heart-valve surgery. The profit margins for these hi-tech procedures may range from 37 percent to 70 percent.

Investigations have shown that such procedures often are unwarranted. They also can be very dangerous for the patient. According to one report, over 90 percent of the million angiograms done each year in this country are uncalled for, and up to 4,500 patients die from the procedure. Nearly 300,000 people undergo balloon angioplasty each year, and from two to four percent die from the procedure or within the following year. It's estimated that 44 percent of heart-bypass patients do not need the operation, and about 5 percent succumb as a result of the surgery.[331]

In many instances less invasive medical treatment, which typically is also less costly, is called for. Indeed, it has been shown that for certain conditions the outcome for patients is often the same whether or not surgery is performed. For example, the number of patients subjected to stroke prevention surgery has risen dramatically. However, when the survival of those who underwent surgery was compared with those patients who only received anti-clogging drugs, the death rates were similar. Ironically, a small number of surgical patients was subjected to an additional risk—the operation itself induced a stroke. Such findings have stimulated *outcomes research*, which attempts to eliminate unnecessary medical procedures by studying what works and what doesn't, and then providing physicians with that information. The results have been encouraging. Physicians have earnestly moved to set guidelines to limit unnecessary operations. Today, nearly every physician specialty group in this country had developed standards of care that clearly specify which patients are proper candidates for which procedures. Also, increasing numbers of medical societies have developed practice guidelines covering a large range of medical procedures. Such guidelines have been found to reduce, if not eliminate, unneeded surgery.[332]

There is some indication that a growing number of patients are becoming victims of the law of induced need, driven by the profit motive of hospitals and physicians. For example, Arizona, in order to promote deregulation, made the decision:

> to abdicate its authority to control the introduction of new open-heart surgery programs. At that time, four Phoenix hospitals provided open-heart surgery. Almost immediately, seven more began programs. A computer-aided study...found that in the first year of deregulation, the local death rate from heart surgery increased by 35 percent. The average cost of the procedure, meanwhile, rose 50 percent(p. 447).

Examples of this kind of risky medicine can be found scattered throughout the nation, as can the overutilization of hi-tech diagnostic equipment as a means of increasing fees. For example, as early as 1992, Broward County, Florida alone had 33 magnetic resonance imaging machines (MRIs), compared with 27 in all of Canada. The point here, however, is not to engage in another expose of the practices and organizations of the major participants in our national health care system. That now occurs with increasing regularity, as evidence mounts "that those who are health care's primary deliverers are also among the greatest threats to its affordability."[333] Rather, it is to emphasize the need for strengthening the *ethical imperative* which should underlie that system. The goal should be to enhance the survival potential of all our citizens, including the poor and the uninsured, who all too often are left unprotected or are denied proper access to the system.

That ethical imperative would, for example, call into question the practice whereby physicians refer patients to treatment facilities in which they have a financial interest. The number and type of tests conducted and the fees charged at these facilities are much higher than at comparable medical units in which physicians do not have such investments. While it is not illegal for physicians to invest in companies that provide medical services and to refer their patients to those facilities, the practice has come under increasing criticism. At the time of this writing, legislation has been introduced to either make it illegal or to regulate it more closely by installing fee caps on various services. As one might expect, such actions have encountered numerous challenges from physicians.

In order to protect the patient, ensure adequate health care at reasonable cost, minimize risks, and provide care designed to promote quality living, reformers have focused on the weaknesses in the current system that have allowed or encourage avarice among medical providers. "New federal laws to curb profitability, software to root out fraud and broad-based research to identify unnecessary medical treatment are aimed at changing the way that doctors practice and ultimately what they're paid."[334] Other innovations, such as health maintenance organizations (HMOs) and preferred-provider networks, which negotiate lower fees based on larger patient groups, are similarly aimed at providing health care protection at reasonable cost. Health care reform is essential if the large and more vulnerable segments of our population are to achieve the same probabilities of wellness and survival that the more privileged currently enjoy.

Corporate Values and Responsibility

The question of ethics is perhaps especially critical at the corporate level. In previous discussion we noted the paramount need for ethical principles that would deter companies from putting profits ahead of keeping people healthy, safe, and alive. Without the application of such principles, backed by severe punishment for those who purposely violate them, life-threatening products can enter the marketplace and place untold numbers of people at risk. Or equally distasteful, certain decisions can be made or practices engaged in which directly or indirectly heighten individuals' vulnerability and lead many to the edge of despair, hopelessness, even suicide. Numerous corporate entities, large and small, can be chosen to illustrate this point and the need for ethical responsibility. Large and small business enterprises eventually interface in various and often complex ways with other industries or governmental agencies. For instance, the makers of silicone breast implants must seek the approval of that product by federal regulators and lobby physicians to promote and support the use of their product. Automobile makers must meet federal safety standards and may lobby politicians to delay the implementation of new standards. Because it is one of the nation's most profitable industries, and because of its pervasive influence on health care, the pharmaceutical industry is selected here to illustrate the importance of an appropriate ethical climate to protect and therefore extend the survival potential of consumers.

The Pharmaceutical Industry. In recent years this industry has come under attack for its aggressive marketing techniques, aimed primarily at physicians but which also permeate nearly every aspect of medical practice, and the excessive costs of its products. In a report on the industry we learn that:

> Drug companies organize "educational symposia" that are actually disguised promotional efforts for their products. They pay for sober-looking "supplements" to respected medical journals and fill those supplements with articles selected and edited to make their products look good. They pay doctors to use drugs in "clinical trials" organized not by drug researchers but by drug marketers. And they offer doctors all sorts of gifts and perks, from ballpoint pens to lavish banquets, and concerts.[335]

The annual cost of these promotional efforts is conservatively estimated to be around $5 billion.

Much of these efforts are aimed at increasing the company's market share of existing products while at the same time achieving greater profits through the sale of higher priced drugs. As the above report notes, while general inflation rose 58 percent between 1980 and 1990, overall health costs rose 117 percent and the cost of drugs increased by 152 percent. The more costly drugs are particularly burdensome to the elderly. While they comprise only 12 percent of the population, they consume 34 percent of prescription drugs. Indeed, surveys reveal that prescription drugs are the single largest out-of-pocket expense for 75 percent of all older Americans, and that 40 percent lack insurance to cover such costs. Consequently, many senior citizens fail to take prescribed drugs because they are too expensive, which practice raises the likelihood of further exacerbation of their medical problems and makes them more susceptible to premature death.

For many years the Food and Drug Administration was unable to cope with the wide-ranging, extravagant, and often questionable promotional practices by the pharmaceutical industry. Here are some examples: sending physicians and their spouses to all-expenses paid "symposia" at Caribbean resorts where their products would be highlighted; offering them frequent flyer mileage for prescribing certain drugs; inviting selected physicians to an expensive restaurant where, prior to eating they would listen to a product presentation and then, at evenings end, be given a money "honorarium" for their time and attention; the placing of "reminder items" (notepads and various trinkets) bearing the company's name in physicians offices and medical centers and distributing same at professional meetings. Sometimes companies provide funds for continuing medical education programs (where required credits can be earned), and then in various ways use those programs as vehicles for product promotion, for instance, by exercising considerable control over the speakers selected, favoring those whose opinions and recommendations were apt to provide positive support for the company line, or by influencing the kinds of instructional materials used. There is evidence that such sponsorship increases sales. Complaints about such practices eventually provoked Senate hearings and eventually prompted the American Medical Association to adopt new codes of ethics that prohibited such lavish incentives.

The result has been some diminution in the more abusive promotional practices, but they have by no means disappeared. For example, at the special dinners, some companies have "complied" with the new AMA rules by substituting gifts of various sorts for the cash honorarium. Many physicians deny that such promotional practices influence or obligate them in any fashion. Yet, the report we are citing here notes that the industry's own market studies show, for example, that 80 percent of dinner meetings subsequently produced increased sales of the target drug among those physicians who were wined and dined. Often these tactics do in fact produce increased sales of higher priced prescription drugs over similar and equally effective, but much lower priced generic equivalents. Ultimately of course, the expenses incurred through various promotional practices are passed on to the consumer, many of whom are increasingly unable to afford the product.

There is growing recognition that the commercially based interdependency of the pharmaceutical industry and science has seriously compromised research, publication, and education. A particularly devious practice of negative marketing disguised as legitimate scientific commentary continues.[336] New rules by the FDA, if enacted and enforced, would go a long way toward rectifying this situation.[337] The medical-academic establishment needs to continue its drive to create a better ethical environment for the profession, one that insures the independence of its members. Hopefully, these complimentary actions "will make the medical marketplace a safer, more honorable one for doctors and patients alike."

Health Education and Life Preservation

Just as individuals can take action to increase the probability of long-term survival, so can society continually seek to promote longevity. This involves, among other things, what health educators refers to as *secondary prevention*, a program of action whose underlying assumption is that early diagnosis and treatment of diseases, and early identification of risk factors that can be controlled, offer the greatest promise for containing the major causes of mortality and disability.[338] There are numerous illnesses which, if diagnosed early and then treated through the application of modern technologies, could spare people from some of the pain and suffering they otherwise experience with later treatment, for example, neoplasms, alcoholism, streptococcal infections, tuberculosis, asthma, irregularities in the functioning of certain organs such as the heart or kidneys, and so on. There are additional conditions whose early recognition can lead to treatment strategies, reorganization of lifestyles, or changes in environmental circumstances that would reduce the otherwise high probability that the people involved would experience a health problem. Included here would be *coronary-risk factors* (cigarette smoking, hypercholesteremia, and hypertension), *accident-risk factors* (alcoholism, epilepsy, and visual defects), *genetic-risk factors* (sickle-cell trait or Tay-Sachs, *lung-risk factors* (smoking, industrial or housing exposures to coal dust, asbestos, mite dust, pollens, exhausts or radiation), *allergic sensitivities* to specific substances, and so forth.[339]

Numerous strategies have been suggested for achieving secondary intervention which are currently available and can be implemented. Among these are multiphasic screening, periodic medical and dental examinations, mass screening for specific conditions, public education regarding early recognition of symptoms and the importance of seeking medical care early for diagnosis of these symptoms, patient education following diagnosis and prescription to improve compliance with therapeutic regimens, genetic counseling, and continuing reinforcement education for the adoption of risk-reduction behavior. A wide range of federal, state, and local government programs has sought to promote the public welfare through minimizing risk factors in virtually all spheres of social life. It is worth repeating, however, that societal efforts to reduce health risks often meet limited success because they are either tempered by political considerations or geared to certain aspects of social life in which decision-making behavior of individuals plays a small role.

Death by Insurance. Citing a study by the Commonwealth Fund, Krugman captures in this title the serious adverse health consequences that lower-income uninsured face in our country. Uninsured adults cut corners on medical care to save money by failing to fill prescriptions and going without preventive care. In his view as well as that of others, the American health care system is in a "gratuitous health crisis" and is "unraveling."[340] These adults are more likely to forego health screenings and less likely to have a regular doctor. The fact that increasingly employers are dropping coverage further exacerbates the problem and makes these people extremely vulnerable to illness and premature demise. The Institute of Medicine estimates that lack of health insurance leads to 18,000 American deaths each year.

Societal incentives must also be constrained by ethical considerations with respect to achieving compliance with health education initiatives while protecting the fundamental rights of citizens. This condition was succinctly articulated in a report to the Department of Health, Education, and Welfare, in which the article's author, cognizant of the relevant ethical issues involved in federal initiatives designed to improve the nation's welfare, recommends that health education be defined as "any combination of learning opportunities designed to facilitate *voluntary* adaptations of behavior which will improve human health" (p. 29). In other words, federal policy must be designed in such a way as to avoid coercing behavior change.

Persuasion versus Coercion: An Ethical Dilemma. Here we touch upon a major dilemma faced by professional health educators, including physicians. In seeking to persuade individuals to alter their lifestyles in order to reduce the risks of illness or premature mortality, they encounter two major ethical principles. Hochbaum[341] describes them as follows:

> We all value the right of the individual to choose his own style of living within his capacity and resources. This implies clearly that, if he chooses to act in ways that endanger his health, fully aware of the risks he takes, he has the right to do so. This individual right is, indeed, the cornerstone of our democratic system. Yet, we all also recognize that every individual has the right to be protected against another individual's actions if these endanger *his* rights, *his* health, and *his* welfare. And we all grant that society has the right to curtail such actions under certain conditions (p.4).

As he sees it, the major dilemma facing health educators in their efforts to get people to adopt voluntarily health habits and practices is deciding which of these principles should predominate, when and under what conditions they should be guided by one or the other, and how far should they go in abiding by one without violating the other beyond justification.

This ethical dilemma presents itself in a wide range of health-related practices whose risks have been open to debate and controversy, for example, the use of chest x-rays, the contraceptive pill, smoking, etc.[342] Some health educators strongly endorse the individual's right to choose his or her lifestyle. They stress the importance of the *principle of informed consent*, whereby consumers are allowed the freedom to choose after they have been given all the information needed to make an intelligent decision. The argument here is that it is a violation of individual rights to force health information or behavior modification on people who do not desire either.

Some health educators take the opposite position—that when it comes to physical and emotional well-being, societal concerns should take precedence over individual prerogatives. They adhere to the position that everyone's rights can be assured only if individuals submit to certain restrictions. That is to say, the actions of individuals cannot be permitted to threaten the health, safety, and welfare of others. When that happens, others have the right to defend themselves. And in such instances health professionals, it is argued, have a duty to identify such actions and prevent them from occurring, either by educational means or by promoting governmental action when necessary.

The conflict between the exercise of individual prerogatives and the desires of others often is related to larger issues of human survival. Consequently, these larger issues not infrequently lead to a confrontation of values. Illustrative here is the case of a married woman with a rare genetic anomaly called **ectrodactyly**, which leads to the partial fusion of finger and toe bones.[343] She already had a 3 year-old daughter born with this same condition when she elected to bear another child with her second husband. They were willing to accept the 50 percent chance that the new child would inherit the disorder, which he did. A television anchorwoman took issue with that decision, voicing personal disapproval, and in her broadcast inviting comments from members of the community, implying that this was not a private affair but one that should concern other citizens. This incensed advocacy groups for the disabled, who charged that the tone of the program was reminiscent of a legislative mood that prevailed earlier in the twentieth century which allowed involuntary sterilization of the mentally retarded in many states. The woman and her husband, along with several national disability advocacy groups, eventually filed a formal complaint with the Federal Communications Commission, which has the power to revoke licenses.

This case raises a number of related life and death issues associated with birth defective children. Some disorders, such as ectrodactyly, are not easily detectable during pregnancy. Others, such as Down syndrome, sickle cell anemia, and cystic fibrosis, can be diagnosed early enough for the parents to decide whether they wish to continue the pregnancy or abort the fetus—never an easy decision. Apparently most couples faced with these circumstances elect to abort. That decision can bring on a confrontation with antiabortionists. In this case, some advocates for the disabled see prenatal screening as a device for identifying the disabled so they can be eliminated.

This raises the controversial issue of *eugenics*—a policy of improving the gene pool by imposing societal control over reproduction. Extreme proponents of this policy take the position that people with certain defective genes should not be allowed to pass them on through their children. The constant battle between pro-abortion and anti-abortion groups, and their solicitation of politicians and courts to support their point of view, reminds us that the potential for state intervention in what has traditionally been considered a private matter is always present.

The tension between individual rights and societal imperatives is exacerbated where scientific information is less than definitive regarding the risks associated with various facets of our life-and-deathstyles. Does taking a daily dose of aspirin prevent heart attacks? Does imbibing a glass of wine each day have positive functions for our well-being? Will megadoses of vitamins enhance our longevity? Are the benefits of irradiated food worth the risk?[344] Is caffeine hazardous to your health or, as one article put it: "To decaf or not to decaf: that is the question..."[345] One could easily construct a rather lengthy list of such questions, as we do in a later chapter, in which the answers are far less definitive than one would desire. In many instances, for example, in the case of irradiated food, the risks remain unknown, despite FDA approval. Similarly, the risks associated with ingesting the caffeine in coffee, tea, and soft drinks remain unclear.

In the early months of 1993, the public was warned, on the basis of limited research findings published in such prestigious journals as *The Journal of the American Medical Association* and *The New England Journal of Medicine*, that men under age 55 with a bald patch on their heads (known as vertex baldness) faced an increased risk of heart attacks, that dreaming predisposes people to heightened cardiac risk, that eating nuts lowers cholesterol levels and hence the risk of heart disease, that men who have undergone vasectomies exhibit an increased risk of developing prostrate cancer, that women taking post-menopausal hormones subsequently experienced serious rates of breast cancer, and, that using hydrogenised margarine is dangerous to one's health! Unfortunately, the majority of people lack training in the scientific method or statistics. Hence, they have "great difficulty interpreting these findings, assessing their validity, recognizing their potential flaws and determining whether a behavioral change is warranted by the evidence."[346] As Brody observes, this steady stream of pronouncements, well publicized through the mass media "can fill otherwise rational people with feelings of panic and paranoia," and lead to "frenetic and pointless changes in habits."[347] Many results from recent medical research are in fact tentative in nature, sometimes run counter to previous findings, often require caveats that diminish their significance and, not infrequently lack additional and strong supporting or explanatory evidence.

The Centenarians. Given the above difficulties, it may come as no surprise to learn that studies of our growing population of centenarians, aimed at discovering the secret of their longevity, often come up with mixed findings. For example, evidence from one recent investigation found that, on the one hand, most of the people who lived to be a 100 years old or more had a close relationship with a spouse, a child, or a nursing-home staff person. Most had an optimistic personality, that is, they evidenced a positive, upbeat outlook on life. Many had avoided caffeine, alcohol and tobacco. As noted in earlier chapters, these are all life-enhancing characteristics. On the other hand, some of these centenarians defied such conventional wisdom all their lives—some regularly consumed alcoholic beverages; others never took medicine. One study of a hundred centenarians who had recovered repeatedly from cancer found that some were chronic worriers, some weighed 235 pounds, and many had spent their lives helping others. When asked why they think they had lived so long, they give varied and often contradictory answers. Health educators would be hard pushed to offer advice on the basis of such comments as: "Keep your feet warm, your head cool, your bowels open, and trust in the Lord."[348]

Findings from a longitudinal study of centenarians reveals certain commonalities that may help explain their longevity and survival. These include a high degree of optimism and a sense of humor, involvement with life, intense interests and activity, resilence in the face of adversity, and an ability to cope with loss. Thus far it appears that these factors, rather than genetics or diet, may play a major role in prolonging the lives of the very old.[349] And it is for these reasons that many of the so-called frail elderly, upon closer scrutiny, often turn out to be not so frail after all. These most recent conclusions run contrary to earlier assumptions, and signal once again the necessity to exercise caution in accepting the latest scientific forecasts at face value.

Final Comment on Informed Consent Paternalistic Legislation

Controversy remains over whether governments should, through legislation, constrain individual or personal risk-taking related to health and mortality. Some view such "paternalistic legislation" as incompatible with democratic values. This position is succinctly summarized by one conservative columnist who argues that "a free people must be be free to be foolish."[350] Others take the opposite position, arguing that legally enacted public health restrictions on life-style choices "are essential to defend the common life and to promote a sense of community."[351] This continuing tug of war between the rights of the individual, on the one hand, and the rights of society on the other, with respect to health issues, is not easily resolved. It often involves important and complex principles related to such notions as social justice, fundamental human rights, and the right to privacy.[352] Conflicts and shifting accomodations characterize efforts to maintain those principles while minimizing the costs to society of voluntary health risks.

Health professionals recognize that while they may view certain behaviors as bringing potentially tragic consequences to a person's well-being, those same behaviors may be so desirable and important to the individual that he or she willingly and gladly accepts the risks. If such a person chooses to ignore health educators persuasive efforts or the information they provide, then, absent a legislated mandate, there is little they can do to effect change without violating the principle of informed consent. Indeed, most are reluctant to do so.

13

Societal Incentives and Survival

The National Agenda

Societal incentives have health consequences and, by implication, survival value. Indeed, it is often the case that a concerted effort at the national level is essential for minimizing the various risk factors which threaten our well-being. The enforcement of drunken driving penalties, the maintenance of air pollution standards, including requirements for minimizing the production of hydrocarbons which damage the ozone layer, and the utilization of catalytic converters and other devices to reduce carbon monoxide emissions, the establishment of mandatory protection from toxic chemicals and other materials, such as asbestos (one of the leading sources of occupational cancer), the enforcement of environmental laws and the punishment of violators, and the dissemination of objective information sources for the consumer—these are all part of a rational strategy to improve human health. Without such a societal effort, the individual initiatives will have limited success. Not that individuals are not important. As one state environmental protection agency administrator was quoted as saying: "It's easy to go out and sue big faceless corporations." However, "Now the problem is us—you, me, our cars, our wood stoves."[353] What is increasingly being suggested is that the achievement of a national health agenda will depend heavily on changes in individual behaviors. But what is the national agenda?

National Goals for Life Preservation

What are the goals of our society to enhance the length and quality of life? The answer to this question is perhaps best found in a series of government reports, mandated by federal legislation. Each of the initial reports was published as a *Prevention Profile* and covered the general state of major health factors in American society. The first such profile, issued in 1980, took cognizance of the growth in knowledge and awareness of how important health promotion and disease prevention could be in reducing unnecessary death and disability in the United States. It also identified a series of prevention indicators and presented current data for each to permit an assessment of where the country stood at the time. A set of improvement goals to be achieved by the next decade was also included.

The most recent edition of the profile, titled *Healthy People 2010: National Health Promotion and Disease Prevention Objectives*, with subsequent *Progress Reports,* continues this effort of monitoring the national progress toward better health.[354] This profile represents a national initiative to improve the well-being of all Americans through prevention, and lays out a set of broad goals for significantly improving the health of the nation by the end of the decade. *Healthy People 2010*, focuses on over twenty priority areas. For each of these areas it specifies the prevalence, goals, and strategies to reduce premature morbidity and mortality in the nation by minimizing or eliminating the risk factors associated with each.

Some of the priority areas, such as the role of physical exercise, smoking and tobacco risks, have already been presented and discussed in previous chapters. In this section I want to take up four particularly pernicious spheres of concern, namely, drug abuse, AIDS, unintentional injuries (accidents), and violent and abusive behavior. These categories directly or indirectly relate to large, at-risk populations, and account for significant numbers of unnecessary deaths each year.

Drug Abuse: An Invitation to Disease and Death

The misuse of drugs has rapidly emerged as a major risk factor in this country. The National Institute on Drug Abuse estimates that over 21 million Americans have tried cocaine, an addictive drug, at least once; and four to five million still use it. The dangerous negative effects of cocaine use on health are intensified when it is consumed through intravenous injections. The sharing of contaminated needles, for example, significantly increases the risk of transmitting the human immunodeficiency virus (HIV). The use of "crack" cocaine has become widespread, especially in urban centers and poverty areas. It appears to be even more addictive than the powdered form of this drug. The rising incidence of developmental disabilities among children of crack-addicted mothers, and the economic burden this places on the health-care system, is of major concern. Cocaine use is on the rise among the younger generation. This trend is particularly alarming, given the potential for addiction. Its costs to society, especially with respect to drug-related crimes, are documented almost daily.

The National Institute on Drug Abuse estimated that over 21 million Americans have also used marijuana in the past year, and nearly 66 million have tried it at least once. Its use is of special concern for the young, since its long-term effects are not fully understood for any age group. Over the short term, marijuana use affects psychomotor skills (for example, driving), especially when used in combination with alcohol. Heroin addiction is thought to be the most serious drug associated with family disorganization and overall crime patterns. In the early 1990's heroin use began rising after many years of decline. The drug problem appears to be worsening, especially in the inner cities of our nation, with a concomitant increase in violent crimes.

The national objectives are aimed at significantly lowering the initiation, prevalence, and intensity of drug use, especially among high risk younger populations, for example, school dropouts and lower income, inner-city youth. The specific goals include education, prevention, and treatment programs designed to reduce drug-related deaths and drug abuse-related hospital emergency department visits. The achievement of these objectives and goals will not be easy. It will take a long-term commitment of people and resources at all levels of government. Without such a commitment, the desired decline in drug use will be extremely difficult to bring about. Perhaps more important, it will require a continued fostering of a social climate that is intolerant of the use of illicit drugs.

> Behavior is strongly influenced by social norms, and norms are shaped, in part, by pubic attitudes and values. They, in turn, affect not only behavior but also legislative and regulatory actions to restrict access to harmful substances and to intensify enforcement of existing laws. Therefore, progress will depend greatly upon maintaining and increasing levels of public education and awareness. (p. 165).

This conclusion is equally applicable to many of the other risk-taking and life-threatening behaviors discussed in this book. A good example of the relationship between behavioral norms and public attitudes, and their connection to other institutional initiatives, was provided in an earlier chapter on changes in smoking behavior. The nearly 180 degree turn in American attitudes toward smoking was accomplished in no small part by a vigorous and persuasive federal public health agenda. Although the problem is complex, similar shifts in norms, attitudes, and behavior can be achieved with regard to drug abuse.

Sexually Transmitted Diseases

General changes in societal mores can have diverse consequences for the quality and length of human life. One example can be seen in the "sexual revolution" which liberalized our norms of intimacy, led to increased sexual contact, and had dire results far beyond gonorrhea and syphilis—both treatable by drug therapy. In recent decades the spectrum of sexually transmitted diseases has expanded dramatically in both complexity and scope. More than 50 such organisms and syndromes are now recognized. Nearly 12 million cases of sexually transmitted diseases occur each year, and close to nine out of ten of these take place among people aged 15 through 29. Its reported that by age 21, about 20 percent of young people have required treatment for one or another form of these diseases.[355] New strains of syphilis and intestinal disorders that are immune to modern drug therapy have emerged because of frequent sexual contact. An increase in hepatitis has brought death to many and a chronic debility to hundreds of thousands. Certain strains of herpes evolved with similar consequences.

The appearance of Acquired Immune Deficiency Syndrome (AIDS) is the latest example of how changes in sexual mores seriously affect life chances. The disease has already been fatal for almost half of the reported cases. Its known incidence continues to rise, and there are perhaps ten times the known number of cases. As so often is the case with life-threatening diseases, young people from socio-economically disadvantaged circumstances run the highest risk of acquiring the virus.[356]

Not only is AIDS one of the leading causes of adult deaths in many undeveloped countries, but it also takes its toll on already burdened health-care systems and on economic development. The more developed countries face similar pressures on their health care system.[357] Many people presently affected by AIDS do not yet know that they have this fatal disease. Indeed, it is quite possible that an individual may unknowingly be infected by more than one type of sexually transmitted disease. Think about this:

> Each sexually active adult can potentially retain infections (apparent or not) acquired from each of his or her previous sexual partners, who may in turn have acquired infections from any of their partners. Under such circumstances one act of extramarital intercourse may expose you to a variety of infections acquired from a large number of different individuals.

There is no handy way of gauging the sexual history of a particular partner. Hence, you generally are not in a position to calculate the degree of risk you are being exposed to:

> Since there is nothing obvious about your partner to indicate the magnitude of the risk you are running, you have to take the information your partner gives you about his or her previous sexual history on trust. Not only is your partner likely to be ill informed, but in the heat of the moment, some partners are also not trustworthy.[358]

While there has been a significant expansion of services for the detection, treatment, and prevention of STD, it is clear that many people who are vulnerable to them are not being effectively served by present programs. Moreover, surveys continue to show that only a minority of persons experiencing multiple sexual partners are consistently using condoms or taking other preventive measures.

The government hopes to reduce significantly the prevalence of all sexually transmitted diseases by encouraging and supporting a variety of programs in different settings across the country. The young are particularly targeted for such efforts. Today, the majority of adolescents have engaged in sexual intercourse by age 20. The risks of early sexual activity include not only unwanted pregnancies and their associated physical and psychosocial problems, but also infection. The most effective means of preventing such problems, of course, would be to delay sexual activity. However, given the current social climate, that does not appear to be a realistic option to most young people. Simplistic solutions are equally unrealistic. Teenage sexual activity is a complex issue, imbedded in family, social, and economic factors. Hence, successful intervention will require the full support and involvement of parents and others who serve in advisory and role-model capacities with teenagers.

A medical cure for AIDS is not yet in sight. As news of its fatal consequences has spread, "safe sex" has quickly become the catch phrase of the day. Translating that slogan into lifestyle behavior changes will be difficult. Unless this is accomplished, however, thousands of lives will be lost unnecessarily. The risk, obviously, just isn't worth it.

Unintentional Injuries and Death

Unintentional injuries (the new terminology for accidents), have accounted for about 100,000 deaths per year. They constitute the fourth leading cause of death in the United States. Up to age 20 unintentional injuries claim more lives than infectious or chronic diseases. Approximately half of these deaths came from motor vehicle crashes. The other causes of accidental death were falls, poisonings, fires, drowning, and residential fires, in that order. In addition, millions of people are seriously incapacitated by unintentional injuries, and many of them suffer lifelong disabilities.

The vulnerability of the young and the older are worth noting here; records show such unintentional events occur in disproportionate numbers among those particular groups, especially young males. Males are more likely to experience unintentional injuries than females, and they are two and a half times more likely to die from them.[359] We have noted early on in this book the activeness, athleticism, adventurousness, and bravado of the young often lead them to engage in risky behavior. This is very much in evidence when one looks at types of accidents. One small example: Each year, skateboard accidents result in 57,000 visits to emergency rooms. The most common injuries involve fractures of the forearm and upper extremities, lacerations, loss of consciousness, loss of teeth, and bone fractures. The most injury-prone among skateboarders are 15-18 year olds.[360]

In the past, the dominant threat to the health of young children came from the major infectious diseases, such as polio, diphtheria scarlet fever, pneumonia, measles and whooping cough. Widespread immunization largely eliminated these threats. Today, unintentional injuries have replaced infectious diseases as the greatest threat to the health of children. Motor vehicle crashes take a particular toll. Interestingly, the National Center for Health Statistics reports that more young school-age children are killed each year in pedestrian accidents than in any other type of accident. It seems that many parents overestimate their young progeny's ability to cross streets alone or to walk to school by themselves, hence placing them unnecessarily in dangerous situations. A significant proportion of injuries to children also occur in or around the home.

Educational efforts aimed at getting parents to recognize their children's developmental limitations and to insure proper supervision, especially of the very young, are part of the national plan to reduce the rate of unintentional injuries. Many injuries can be and are being prevented through improved safety measures, including swimming pool and spa covers and childproof enclosures; child-resistant packaging for prescription drugs and some other hazardous materials; safer playground equipment; and smoke detectors.[361] With greater use of protective child carriers in cars, and an increased and consistent employment of seat belts, that death and injury from accidents can be significantly reduced.

Controlling Violent and Abusive Behavior

Someone once asserted that violence is as American as apple pie. There is considerable truth in that statement. Government data show that child abuse and spouse abuse, and other forms of intrafamilial violence continue to threaten the lives of thousands of individuals, often resulting in lethal consequences. The United States ranks first among the industrialized nations of the world in violent death rates. The number of deaths caused by violent and unintentional misuse of firearms surpasses the *combined* total of other modern nations. Suicide is the third leading cause of death among people aged 15 through 24, and homicide is the leading cause of death for blacks aged 15-34. The toll in terms of years of *potential life lost*,[362] as well as injury-related deaths and long-term disabilities, is staggering. "It appears that violence has become the response of first recourse in many cases of emotional and mental distress and interpersonal conflict, as well as a tool of premeditated criminal acts." (p.226).

Because it takes a huge toll in terms of morbidity and mortality, and at enormous economic cost, the national agenda now defines violent and abusive behaviors as a priority public health problem. It recognizes that since many violent behaviors resulting from stress are affected by socioeconomic conditions, ameliorative strategies must go beyond the health care system or the criminal justice system to include a variety of societal sectors. The agenda delineates a specific set of objectives for reducing the problem in six key areas: homicide and assaultive violence, domestic violence, child abuse, sexual assault, suicide, and firearm injury.

Deadly Firearms. It is not my intent to cover all these in this book. The topic of homicide has been widely researched, and those findings could easily fill a several volumes. Rather, I choose to focus on one area in particular, namely the growing threat posed by the widespread prevalence and use of firearms. In 1990 alone, nearly 20,000 persons between the ages of 1 and 34 died as a result of a firearm injury.[363] Today, one's survival all too often depends on the whim of someone, distressed or otherwise, pointing a handgun, rifle, or even an assault weapon in his direction.[364] The weapons most often employed in homicides are firearms, usually handguns, followed by knives. Firearms are both the most lethal and the most common instrument used for suicide and homicide, accounting for approximately 60 percent of these violent deaths each year.[365] The Los Angeles riots in 1992 demonstrated all too clearly to the nation, via television in living color, how well armed some neighborhood citizens were, and how quickly they were prepared to use their weapons. It was a vivid commentary on the state of the nation and its inability to preserve law and order—and life.

There are now over 200 million privately owned guns in the United States, with manufacturers pouring four to five million more new weapons onto the market each year. This massive presence of weapons has given rise to the fear among many that we have become "a nation bleeding from an oversupply of fire-power."[366] About half of all households in the country own at least one gun. It is important to note in this connection that over time, the type of guns that Americans buy and the reasons for buying them have both undergone change. Up through the 1950s shotguns and rifles, long associated with rural life, hunting, and pest control, were the weapons of choice, followed by handguns. Sales of all three types were less than two million annually. Starting in the 1960s, however, the market was transformed as a result of various social upheavals involving assassinations, riots, drug abuse, and soaring crime rates. Subsequently the sales of new guns rose steadily so that today every other weapon sold is a handgun. Several million used guns also change hands each year, although the exact number is almost impossible to determine, since most such private transfers escape federal record-keeping rules.

Guns are in abundance, and can easily and illegally be purchased out on the streets of our cities, no questions asked.[367] Incidents of young teenagers showing up at schools to settle arguments, or to protect themselves, or for other reasons, are just one reflection of the easy access to weapons in today's society. The availability of handguns to urban high school students is particuarly pervasive. Apparently they can acquire such weapons with little difficulty.[368] In increasing numbers teenage males and young men, as well as women, are becoming victims of the violent use of firearms. Indeed, in the United States the leading cause of death among both black and white teenage males is gunshot wounds.[369] Moreover, with so many American households now containing one or more weapons, the potential for accidental killings is increasingly present. Accidental shooting deaths of very young children are particularly tragic. Data complied by the Center to Prevent Handgun Violence, a not-for-profit agency in Virginia, show that nearly 300 children under the age of 14 are killed in firearm accidents each year. This amounts to more than 16 percent of all accidental deaths involving a gun. In recent years, several states have passed controversial legislation which makes adults who negligently store weapons within the reach of children criminally liable if a child is injured or killed. Opponents of such laws have argued that they do more harm than good by compounding the tragic suffering of the adults and families involved. Supporters, on the other hand, argue that enforcement of these laws is essential in order to protect children from the carelessness with which adults sometimes treat deadly weapons.[370]

Over time the handgun of choice has also shifted, from revolvers to semi-automatic pistols, which can hold many more cartridges. They are spring loaded from a magazine into the firing chamber with each shot. The magazines allow easy and quick reloading. These are a far cry from the standard six-cylinder revolver of the past, and more dangerous.

As stated earlier, firearms fatalities are only one aspect of the larger issue of violence, in both its fatal and nonfatal outcomes, as a public health problem. In fact, given their much greater incidence, "nonfatal outcomes of self-directed and interpersonal violence may represent a problem of even greater social, economic, and political importance."[371] In this section, however, we have focused on fatal results with respect to firearm use. If such homicidal outcomes are to be prevented or reduced, if not eliminated, a range of public health strategies will be necessary, including programs to decrease the cultural acceptance of violence, and the teaching of nonviolent conflict resolution skills.

Changing attitudes of the public toward the possession and use of weapons is no simple matter. This is highlighted by the ongoing controversy over gun control. Despite considerable evidence that gun control laws can lead to sharp declines in gun related deaths, legislation is strongly resisted by many citizens and groups.[372],[373] The best known and most powerful organization that opposes such legislation is the National Rifle Association. It consistently argues that "guns don't kill people, people kill people." To which supporters of such legislation retort, "But people with guns kill people."[374] Some argue that little headway will be made in reducing the availability and access to handguns and other weapons until that controversy and related issues are resolved. The former Surgeon General of the United States and other health officials have proposed that the right to own or operate a firearm carry with it the same type of responsibilities required to operate motor vehicles. Specifically, they suggest that the owner and operator of a firearm meet the following criteria:

- be of a certain age and physical\mental condition;
- be required to demonstrate knowledge and skill in proper use of that firearm;
- be monitored in the firearm's use; and
- forfeit the right to own or operate the firearm if these conditions are abrogated.

These restrictions would apply uniformly to all firearms and nationwide though a national system of gun registration and licensing, without exception.[375]

Others suggest that the implementation of a broad range of measures are necessary, including parental supervision to prevent immediate access to weapons and ammunition by children, educational campaigns designed to reduce the romanticization of guns and to communicate the relative risks and benefits of keeping firearms in the home, so that people can make more informed decisions. Still others argue that more stringent regulation and monitoring of gun purchases, and legislative measures with respect to waiting periods or prescribing mandatory jail terms for illegal carrying of firearms, could contribute to the alleviation of this widespread problem. Unless these or other agendas are implemented to safeguard the public's health, firearms are likely to replace motor vehicles as our leading cause of traumatic death.[376]

Summary

This chapter has emphasized that life patterns of mortality are not randomly distributed. They reflect an array of factors that underscore the close link between societal conditions and their impact on the individual. Technological and social changes can be profound in promoting or threatening life chances. Our discussion of major health and mortality topics leads to the conclusion that there is still a great need to develop and implement a societal commitment to longevity and improvement of the quality of life. Such a commitment would be a significant impetus in achieving the overall goal that the government has established for enhancing our survival potential by reducing the risks of premature death.

14

Population Growth

Threat to the Environment and Human Survival

The unchecked multiplication of people may prove to be the most urgent and immediate threat to the planet and hence to human survival. The geometrical rapidity of population growth has been well documented. It took all of recorded history for the world to reach 1 billion people by the year 1830. It only took the next hundred years to reach the 2 billion mark, and a mere 30 years to arrive at 3 billion. We are currently adding nearly a billion people each decade. By the end of the twentieth century, world population reached more than 6 billion. By 2025, the number of humans inhabiting the earth may be more than 50% more than they currently are. This "population explosion," has numerous demographic and societal consequences, not the least of which are the exacerbation of environmental degradation and the depletion of resources. Left unchecked, these conditions pose serious threats to governmental institutions and national economies and, eventually, to human survival.

Such growth endangers the environment in numerous ways, since each new person needs some portion of the earth's resources for food, shelter, energy, and water. Hence:[377]

- Each additional person adds an increment to the demand on the environment, making the situation a little worse.

- Each person's demand is multiplied to varying degrees by the person's affluence and by the environmental impact of technologies involved in production and consumption.

- The high population density of large cities, resulting partly from high birthrates, overwhelms water supply, sanitation, and waste disposal systems.

- The rapid pace of population growth leaves little time to promote environmental safeguards and to introduce new technologies. Solving environmental problems is more difficult and more expensive when populations grow too quickly.

- The steadily increasing burden of growing population can eventually overload natural systems, causing their collapse.

These potential outcomes are especially real for those living in the less developed and often poorest countries of the world. Overpopulation in many of these places is damaging the environment in ways that increasingly threatens human survival, as well as plant and animal species, many of which are disappearing annually. More than half of the developing countries may be unable to feed their populations from their own lands.

Deforestation. The situation with respect to the world's forests illustrate the severity of social and environmental problems that can be provoked by the presence of too many people. Forests account for almost 30 percent of the earth's total land area. Nations are becoming increasingly aware that well managed natural and man-made forests can provide a wide range of economic, social, and environmental benefits to improve human welfare. Unfortunately, in many places the integrity and stability of forest ecosystems are being threatened.[378] For example, seventy percent of so-called Third World families depend solely on wood for their fuel. To meet that need, they are rapidly eliminating what is already in many areas a scarce resource. Hence, it has been estimated that by the end of this decade almost half of the world's people (three of every five people in developing countries) will lack sufficient fuelwood.

Massive amounts of topsoil erosion take place in part because of deforestation. Twenty-five billion tons of arable topsoil vanishes from the world's cropland each year. Deforestation in the tropics alone is now estimated at nearly 20 million hectares annually, an area almost equivalent to Britain or Uganda. Among the unwelcome outcomes of such decimation are a loss of biodiversity, possible global climate change, degradation of watersheds, and desertification.[379] The depletion of forests together with land degradation contributes to the rapidly growing disparity between the Earth's dwindling resources and the number of people sharing them.[380] This situation can threaten subsistence levels and result in widespread poverty, hunger, and starvation among some of the world's demographic subgroups, especially among developing nations.

These negative consequences of degraded forest land also highlight the fact that, under the demanding press of ever-growing numbers, overpopulated regions and countries around the world will be less and less able to uphold the principle of *sustainable development*, that is, "meeting people's current needs while preserving nature's productive capacity for the future."[381] What this means is balancing conservation and development goals or objectives. While this is a complex, difficult, often costly task, and one that must be carried out within and across nations, it is absolutely essential if natural resources are to be protected and preserved for the generations to come.

The lengthy litany of potential catastrophes inherent in unchecked human growth can be frightening. Even rational scientific discourse about the problem can quickly take on the aura of depressing doomsday projections. Only a few of these potential disasters are presented here.[382]

Water. Population pressures increasingly threaten the pool of available fresh water. Less than one percent of the earth's water is available for human consumption, and much of that is unsafe to drink due to widespread pollution. Expanding concentrations of people reside near the world's ocean coasts, and feeding them has led to dangerous levels of overfishing, thereby taxing the ocean's productive capacity.[383] Moreover, natural ecosystems are being damaged by heavy pollution (our oceans have become garbage dumps for waste and sewage) and by dredging and filling of wetlands to make room for additional development. Over half of all Americans live within 50 miles of a coastal shoreline.[384] In short, burgeoning human numbers can lead to declining resources, creating a situation which, if left unchecked, can in time place both people and planet in mortal danger.

In the view of most experts, this situation can best be prevented through the implementation of effective and comprehensive family planning programs designed to achieve population stabilization, which in turn helps to improve the economy. Unfortunately, access to such programs is often limited. The World Fertility Survey estimates that some 500 million women who desire and need family planning information lack either the information or the means to obtain it. The result is a considerable number of unnecessary maternal and child deaths each year "from pregnancies which are too early, too late, too many and too close together, as well as from abortions."[385]

The Overconsumption Problem.

The dangers of overpopulation, however, are not to be found simply in numbers of people. Overconsumption, made possible through technological innovations and expansion, also plays a significant role. Industrialized nations represent only 20 percent of the world's people, but *consume* 80 percent of the world's resources.

Americans reading about the potential "population crisis" exhibit relatively little concern. Many are not even convinced that there is such a crisis. But there is little question that we are the world's greatest consumers. "By the age of 75, a child born in the United States today will have produced *52 tons* of garbage, consumed 10 million *gallons* of water, and used 5 *times* more energy than a child born in the Third World."[386] As other developed and developing countries modernize, they too tend to increase their consumption of resources. The world's resources, of course, are not unlimited, and we are rapidly exhausting those which remains. For example:

> Nearly all of the world's commercial power is derived from fossil fuels—oil, coal, and natural gas. Currently, the world uses in one year an amount of fossil fuel that took nature roughly one millon years to produce. At current consumption levels, and assuming no population increase, the readily accessible supplies of oil will be exhausted within 40 years, and natural gas, in 60 years. Coal supplies will last much longer—for hundreds of years at current consumption rates. Switching to more coal, however, is likely to worsen air pollution and hasten the onset of global warming.[387]

Widescale conversion from oil to alternative energy sources such as hydropower and solar power, worldwide conservation efforts, the development of more energy-efficient technologies, and restrictions on various expanding human activities that contaminate and destroy the atmosphere and the earth, have become all too apparent essentials for sustaining life.

For the planet and its people to survive, environmental protection will have to be given a much higher priority than it currently receives. In a very real sense, time for corrective action may be running out. In a 1992 report it was argued that:

> If we do nothing between now and the year 2000 to counteract current trends, it will take several centuries for the world's forest cover to be restored, as much as 1,000 years for depleted topsoil to be replenished, and several thousand years or more to bring the earth's climates back to today's conditions. Species made extinct and aquifer (underground water deposits) that are polluted will be lost forever.[388]

It is generally agreed that fertility decisions designed to reduce population growth can play a crucial role in efforts to avoid such scenarios from coming to pass. Reduced birthrates can provide some breathing room for correcting prior environmental neglect and give nature time to renew the land, forests, and fresh water. Achieving smaller family sizes now can make significant differences for future demands on the environment. If a woman has two children, and each of them and their children has two children, she will have eight great-grandchildren. However, if a woman has four children, and so do her children and their children, then she will have sixty-four great-grandchildren. This is a rather dramatic difference. Reduced birthrates hold out the hope of achieving a better balance between meeting people needs and the exploitation of natural resources.

Demographers estimate that under various natural and human corrective actions the population explosion could run its course by the end of the 21 century. At that time the number of people on the earth will range between eleven and thirteen billion. Whether the planet can support such a hugh population is unknown, though it is possible to conceive of a world in which there are too many people to be supported by the available environmental resources. Many experts suggest that ten billion people may be the maximum that could be supported comfortably. Still others believe that the world's basic biological systems are incapable of maintaining such numbers and predict that long before we approach the ten billion figure major system failures will occur. Whatever the peak carrying capacity of the earth might be, there is little disagreement that a more concerted effort to stabilize population growth is desirable. Indeed, that effort is essential for maintaining the environment and the human condition as we know it.[389]

Conclusion

In the final analysis, survival of the species will depend on the willingness of the world community to commit to a global strategy to preserve a healthy planet through sustainable management of its varied and sensitive ecosystems.[390] A clear and unrelenting *active* commitment to such a strategy on the part of individuals and nations will be difficult to achieve. It will require the pursuit of a new global "ethic of survival," in which the hierarchy of values and priorities for living are rearranged in order to halt the growing threat to mankind.[391] The continuing challenge of this new ethic will be to resolve the inevitable conflicts that arise between the exercise of personal autonomy, and the requirements essential for maintaining civilization. That challenge will require establishing an acceptable balance between individual prerogatives and the vital needs of society.

It may also mean launching an "environmental revolution," one which would entail drastic restructuring the global economy (including moving away from the use of fossil fuels), major shifts in human reproductive behavior (stabilizing population size in order to reestablish the balance between people and the natural systems upon which they depend), and dramatic changes in values and lifestyles.[392] The proponents of this agenda argue that, unlike the long historical periods required to effect the changes wrought by the Agricultural and Industrial revolutions, the Environmental Revolution must take place within the next few decades in order to avoid widespread catastrophic outcomes. However, given the immense worldwide economic and social transformations called for by this revolution, as well as the essential shifts in values and lifestyles that would be required, it is doubtful that its overall goal of "building an environmentally sustainable future" will be achieved within that time frame. While many encouraging actions have already been taken by various nations, so much more remains to be done.

> If the Environmental Revolution is to succeed, it will need the support of far more people than it now has. In addition to overcoming vested interests, it must also overcome human inertia. Up until now the Environmental Revolution has been viewed by society much like a sporting event—one where thousands of people sit in the stands watching while only a handful are on the playing field actively attempting to influence the outcome of the contest. Success in this case depends on erasing the imaginary sidelines that separate spectators from participants so we can all get involved. Saving the planet is not a spectator sport.[393]

15

Living Is Risky

Americans have become increasingly responsive to health information and are incorporating that information into life saving risk assessment orientations. These orientations are, in turn, encouraged by the activities of a variety of local, state, and federal agencies, and involve risk management programs designed to ensure better health. The Centers for Disease Control, for example, are directly concerned with protecting and promoting good health. Their research and reports concerning such topics as cholesterol and nitrates have helped alter our eating habits. The American Cancer Society's promotion of an anticancer diet which stresses high-fiber foods has similarly prompted many people to change their consumption habits.

It is important to reemphasize, however, that without some modification in individual behavior, the societal effort will have only limited success. Indeed, there is a widespread feeling that perhaps the best hope for achieving increased survival may lie in the voluntary efforts derived from personal choice. We have noted that there is a countless array of options people can take to increase their life chances. Growing acceptance of the scientific evidence of a connection between such habits as smoking and certain health hazards often has a "ripple effect," in that it starts people thinking about their survival potential.[394] The alteration of those habits of our lifestyles which have deleterious consequences is increasingly recognized as one of the major direct routes to a long and relatively risk-free existence. To be most effective, these changes must be accompanied by a concomitant shift in attitudes which support a *rational* approach to daily living.

Perhaps "rational" should be underscored, since some people, faced with almost daily revelations about things that potentially impair their health, may react either by dismissing their significance altogether, or becoming health conscious in the extreme. Several newspaper columnists, perhaps reflecting these possible public reactions, have commented on the surfeit of daily or weekly disclosures and the mounting tabulation of newly discovered risks surrounding our daily living. A widely read editorialist titled one of his newspaper columns *Almost Everything Can Kill Us*. He is chagrined by the growing list of things that health authorities recommend we avoid, many of which he describes, and comments: "There are times, as all of us in this health-conscious society are aware, when it appears that everything is bad for us and nothing at all is good for us." He noted one report which listed 200 things that various authorities have warned us to avoid because in one way or another they are bad for the health of *some* people in *some* circumstances, including: tobacco, fresh air (cited by two physicians who found that breathing too much of it can cause insomnia and nightmares), air conditioning (because a leading microbiologist indicated that it could cause asthma in some people), living too close to jet airports, overexposure to anesthetics (supposedly makes female nurses more susceptible to childbirth problems, some over-the-counter antacids (which may complicate kidney problems), apricots and cherries (they are related to cyanide), aquariums (they often contain a bacterium that can cause skin trouble), asphalt road surfaces (a United Nations committee says they may contain cancer-causing agents), certain bleaches (the American Medical Association states that they will react on the elastic in underwear so as to cause rashes), books (a study found that library workers can contract the viral infection known as "historians lung"), Brussels sprouts, cabbage, cauliflower, and collard greens (all supposedly inhibit iodine intake and hence contribute to goiters), chlorine, chromium, cola, color TV sets, cranberries, cats, dogs, eggs, electric shavers, flea collars and fluorescent lights, fluoride, fly ash, formaldehyde, fungicides, gas stoves, gasoline, glue and golf balls. Numerous items in the list are said by some investigator somewhere to be associated with cancer, including bread mold, black pepper, hair dyes, hot soup, leeks, the lack of iodine, synthetic fibers in leisure suits (because when affected by perspiration release a cancer-causing gas), lettuce (found to have carcinogenic traces), migratory birds mushrooms (contains certain carcinogenic compounds), olive oil, and peanut butter. Additional potential hazards to one's health come from the use of lawn mowers, tricycles and swimming pool slides, as well as kissing (transmits mononucleosis), too much orange juice (contributes to decay of tooth enamel), etc.. The columnist finally threw in the towel, shouting: "Enough, enough! Summon the hearse, and let us die in peace."[395]

Another columnist similarly discussed a lengthy litany of dangerous dietary habits uncovered by science and decries "the brain-numbing pile of research data thrown upon us by people telling us what to eat and drink, do or not do, if we are to have any hope of living a long and healthy life."[396] He, like many, is often irritated and confused by the sometimes ambiguous or contradictory evidence offered by the lifestyle researchers. He, like many, laments over the numerous and favorite things he will have to eliminate from his lifestyle in order to minimize risks and live a long and healthy life, such as "those delightful fat-marbled steaks, or thick pork chops, that I put on my grill; fewer cheese omelets that are wolfed down with pork sausages or bacon." His list of do-nots, drawn from various reports, included the avoidance of many of his favorite meals which contained saturated fats—eggs benedict, liver with crisp bacon, polish sausage slices in spaghetti sauce, coffee and caffeine, artificial sweeteners, smoking, etc., etc. He was particularly chagrined over the fact that the recommendations from the experts would often be contradictory, for example, those regarding milk, or the water we drink. Beneath the surface of his not-so-tongue in cheek commentary one almost hears the familiar complaint that having to change habitual and pleasurable consumption patterns "takes all the fun out of life."

Indeed, one could easily get depressed from reading the litany of possible catastrophes that surround our daily living. A cursory perusal of my files reveals that in recent years we have been warned by the mass media of the following presumed dangers, often extrapolated from less than convincing research evidence, and often based upon animal studies only: taking a shower (chemicals in the water quietly transform into vapors which expose us to chemical concentrations ten times greater than we would get by drinking the water), handling money (over 10 percent of all coins and more than 40 percent of paper money carry infectious organisms), teeth whiteners (the primary chemicals used in most whiteners could damage mouth tissue and tooth pulp, and may enhance the effect of carcinogens), tooth fillings containing mercury (it can escape from the fillings, enter body tissues and impair organ function—at least in animals), drinking from lead crystal glasses or ingesting wine stored in crystal decanters (can lead to lead poisoning or trigger gout), living too close to utility power lines (exposes you to health damaging electromagnetic fields, supposedly capable of suppressing the immune system and causing leukemia, lymphoma, and brain cancer), electric blankets, heating pads, and water beds (women who use them apparently suffer more miscarriages than those who don't; ditto for those women who work in front of a computer video-display terminal), frequent flying (increases cancer risk because of higher level of radiation at higher altitudes), dry cleaning your clothes (the most commonly used chemical, perchoroethylene, is dangerous—it pollutes water, may damage the ozone layer, and may cause cancer, and using cellular telephones (some believe that electromagnetic energy radiating from these phones either causes or accelerates cancer growth).

Perhaps nothing quite tops the pronouncement, carried in newspapers and magazines across the country, that, as one headline put it, "Getting Out of Bed May Be The Riskiest Act of the Day."[397] A study completed at the Deaconess Hospital in Boston discovered that the risk of dropping dead from a heart attack is twice as high in the few hours after arising in the morning than at any other time of day. We are not told, of course, how one is to avoid this heightened possibility of a heart attack. Sooner or later, we must face this daily peril of arising. After having read about this, I found myself, at least for a short while, consciously getting out of my bed in a slow and deliberate manner, spending a few moments sitting up, all the while listening for any signal of impending cardiac arrest.

In many circumstances, the presumed threat to one's survival becomes impossible to counter. For example, one study reported that *dreaming* may be hazardous to a person's health.[398] It seems that the time during sleep when dreams occur an individual experiences considerable tension, which sets the so-called sympathetic nervous system into motion. This system, designed to prepare the body for emergencies, induces a rapidly accelerated heart rhythm and rising blood pressure, as stress hormones prepare the body for the fight or flight response. It was found that the sympathetic nervous system was twice as active during dream periods as is normal when people are awake. This led the researchers to speculate that such inner turmoil may trigger heart attacks, especially among those with heart trouble. Even if such speculation is eventually confirmed, there is little that one can do about dreaming!

Just when we think we have exhausted the deadly litany of environmental risks a new one appears. According to a recent report people who choose to be cremated rather than buried pose a serious health hazard.[399] Apparently as the corpse burns, the mercury in tooth fillings vaporizes into a highly toxic gas. This gas, which escapes through the chimney, is capable of causing neurological and kidney damage. It is unclear whether the mercury concentrations around crematoria exceed safe air standards. Mercury toxicologists, however, point out that the vapor can remain in the atmosphere for months.

While one can avoid crematoria and its toxic emissions, some threats to our existence are impossible to dismiss. Boston researchers reported finding a significant relationship between a person's height and the probability of having a heart attack, with men of short stature facing the greatest danger.[400] Men who were 5 feet 7 inches or shorter had a 60 percent greater risk of developing a first heart attack than men 6 feet 1 inch or taller. Apparently the shorter men are more prone to heart attacks because their coronary arteries are narrower than those of tall men and thus more vulnerable to damage from buildup of fatty deposits or blood clots. More short men in the study were overweight, had higher cholesterol levels and high blood pressure. However, analysis revealed that height alone was a major contributor and was independent of other risk factors, such as frequency of exercise, cholesterol level, smoking and age. Does this mean that small men are doomed to face cardiac arrest or that tall men are resistant to such experience? Obviously not. But such findings typically trigger a new round of worry over the latest threats to our well-being.

The litany of presumed hazards continues unabated through nutritional bulletins headlined in our newspapers and magazines. For instance, the public has been warned via the mass media, by what one writer terms the "food police," that excess iron in the blood might cause heart disease, that the consumption of milk might trigger diabetes and allergies, and that using margarine could raise blood cholesterol levels. "And then there's the never-ending saga of oat bran—does it or doesn't it help lower cholesterol?—regardless of whether or not lowering cholesterol is a good thing. The price to be paid for such hyper vigilance to nutrition news is utter confusion."[401] Provocative media pronouncements, often based upon a single study, are perplexing because they often contradict conventional wisdom and heretofore accepted recommendations on eating healthfully. It is, therefore, worth remembering that the core principles of nutrition for disease prevention have remained the same since they were first developed. In fact, the majority of experts are in agreement that "front-page nutrition news tends to obscure an otherwise consistent message of what makes up a healthy diet," including the longstanding advice to "choose lean meats and low-fat dairy products, eat more fruits, vegetables and grains, and cut back on fat wherever you can."[402] Taking news flashes about nutrition research with a grain of salt if not a healthy dose of skepticism may help allay unnecessary concern and anxiety. One nutritionist offers this sage advice for minimizing overreactions to the latest nutritional news. "Before the headlines send you on a search-and-destroy mission in your refrigerator, go beyond the headlines and read or listen to the story. Chances are, somewhere in there it will say: 'Don't change your diet just yet. More research is needed.'"[403]

Some Comic Relief

Not surprisingly, those that dismiss the significance of many health risks often use humor as a weapon to combat their own anxieties about disease, illness, death and dying. Humorist Lewis Grizzard, for example, titled one of his pieces *Things That Go Bump In The '80s* and *another What You Don't Know Won't Kill You,*[404] both comically describing all the things that frightened him (and us) as a result of the risk-taking information disseminated through the mass media. He not-so-jokingly questions whether increasing public awareness of the potential health hazards associated with certain kinds of cholesterol in our food, pesticide residues on our salads, AIDS, the warming of the planet, asbestos, nuclear leaks, and so on, is altogether beneficial. He contends that the daily or weekly assault of ominous headlines regarding life and death matters tends to overwhelm and frighten us, and produces levels of stress not experienced by prior generations. In his partially jocular rationale, he suggests we all would be better off if the press kept certain such matters quiet. In other words he, and I suspect many others, would rather not know about health risks at all.

This might be termed the *ostrich approach* to living. The ostrich supposedly buries his head in the sand, thereby rendering him oblivious to threats from predators and other hazards in the surrounding environment. If anything subsequently happens which shortens his life, it isn't his fault. After all, he wasn't aware of impending danger and, therefore, had no control of his eventual demise.

The Devil Made Me Do It

Admittedly, the poor ostrich does have less dominion than humans over the environment. But humans can exercise considerable caution and control and, therefore, can be held accountable for their actions. Flip Wilson, a one-time popular television comedian, would often have skits in which he would attempt to avoid culpability for this or that embarrassing behavior or situation by offering that now familiar line—"the devil made me do it." Often, those seeking to avoid accountability delude themselves by invoking the oft-repeated statement: "I can't help myself," as an excuse for failed attempts to amend unhealthy lifestyles. Some have contended that such attempts at exoneration constitute a sort of "new obscenity" in which humans are perceived as organisms devoid of free will and, therefore, are unable to resist powerful biological and social forces.[405] The result is a "I can't help myself" stance, reminiscent of our earlier discussion of fatalism, which ultimately leads to avoidance of individual responsibility. People holding such a view often consider their inability to quit self-destructive habits as reflecting forces beyond their control. For example, they tend to define dangerous habits as addictions over which they lack the power to overcome. Hence, they regard any efforts to alter their life-reducing behaviors, for example, by exercising self-discipline or moderating their bad habits, as futile.

Compulsions and Addictions: Risk Denial?

In recent years a widening spectrum of compulsive behaviors and addiction problems have been portrayed as biologically rooted diseases whose treatment lie
beyond individual control. This model has been criticized by some because it
conveys a harmful message to abusers which not only excuses irresponsibility, but
also indoctrinates them with the idea they're helpless and sick. Concern is being
expressed over "society's willingness to expand the definition of addictive disease
beyond substance abuse to include a host of excessive behaviors—ranging from
shopping to promiscuity—and clinicians' readiness to treat what may be social
and willpower problems as medical disorders instead."[406] The fear is that such
disease-oriented programs may have the unanticipated consequence of absolving
people of the personal liability for their habits.[407]

Some people, then, choose to ignore all risks because they believe they lack the
prerogative to eliminate them. In the view of many others, however, those who
excuse their bad habits and addictions as a result of uncontrollable forces are simply seeking to avoid accountability for their actions. Wilbanks, for example, takes
the position that people *choose* to become addicts and that drug addiction (and,
indeed, other so-called addictions) is primarily a moral rather than a medical
problem. Hence, he is convinced that the most effective treatment we can offer
people is to hold them responsible for their behavior. In line with that position,
which represent one polar end of a continuum of perspectives ranging from fatalism at one extreme to total personal accountability at the other, he advises that
"the next time someone tells you, 'I can't help myself,' don't believe it. And do
the person a favor—say so."[408]

Some of these risk-denial attitudes may reflect an unanticipated paradox.
Intensified efforts to educate the public about an ever-widening range of potential hazards may reach a point where the sheer volume of information becomes
overwhelming. This, in turn, can lead some people to screen out further warnings, thereby increasing their vulnerability to current and future hazards. Given
that they feel inundated with voluminous dangerous-to-your-health information,
it is understandable that some people may desire, or actually seek to relieve stress
in their lives by dismissing the realities of life-threatening elements in the environment.

The other extreme reaction is to become overly health conscious. In the face of
widespread threats to their survival potential, some persons will try to avoid *all*
risks, including those associated with normal living. They may live out their lives
in total isolation while waiting for the nuclear war, or they might ingest daily

mega doses of vitamins to combat inevitable aging and its associated morbidities. Whatever their strategy, the obsession with avoiding all risks can be a risk itself because the long-term consequences of many of these practices are not well known.[409] For example, large doses of some vitamins are benign; but the effects of others, such as mega doses of Vitamin A, can be deadly. Health extremists seem to presume that if they can avoid all risks, they can live longer than average.

Sometimes an over concern with the potential risks of daily living can lead to *nosophobia*, that is, a morbid dread of disease, which can border on psychosis. Indeed, some argue that due to widespread publicity given to the rising crescendo of potential threats to our well-being, nosophobia has become a national psychosis, illustrated by recent panics about cancer-causing chemicals in food. The public fear over the use of the pesticide Alar (technical name, *daminozide*), commonly sprayed on apple orchards, is one such example. This plant-growth regulator is used to keep ripening apples on the tree. It also acts to keep the fruit firm and red during the post-harvest storage, thereby reducing spoilage. When it was reported that high doses of Alar caused cancer in laboratory animals, the public panicked by throwing away or avoiding apples and apple products. Some cities rushed to remove apples from grocery shelves and school cafeterias. Various consumer groups and environmental activists, such as the Natural Resources Defense Council (NRDC) called for an immediate ban on this pesticide. In the latter instance, for example, it was noted that a carcinogen byproduct of Alar, identified as UDMH, was released whenever apples were cooked to make juices and sauces, and that:

> …the risk from UDMH has many features that make it less acceptable to consumers than other, far larger risks that we live with daily. It's not like smoking, a risk people more or less consciously choose. It's not like driving a car, whose riskiness is largely under one's own control. It's not like radon gas seeping through the basement floor or aflatoxin in peanuts, since UDMH is in foods by human hands, not Nature. It's not like prescription drugs, whose users sometimes bear risks but reap the benefits as well. An unlike many risks, this one falls disproportionately on children.[410]

It was for these reasons that the editors of *Consumer Reports* found the presence of Alar in foods to be intolerable and called for its ban.

The fact of the matter is that many foods contain chemicals that, *if* administered in *high* doses, will cause cancer in lab animals including table pepper, sugar, calcium, mushrooms, peanuts, soy sauce, even bread. Humans, of course, do not normally ingest such dangerously high concentrations. In this connection, it has been contended that:

> trace levels of pesticide residue have never been implicated in ill health in any human being, ever. There has never been a documented case of ill health related to pesticide residues from regulated, approved use of pesticides...If people want to extend their longevity, they should stop throwing out wholesome food and focus on real risks...smoking, alcohol abuse, illicit drug use, not eating a moderate diet, failing to use lifesaving technology—like seat belts or smoke detectors.[411]

While industry experts, scientists, and consumer advocates argue as to where the truth lies in such matters, the public often becomes confused and frightened.[412] When people feel threatened they often behave irrationally. Not infrequently, common sense becomes a casualty. As just noted, in moments of fear, they may throw out the apples which are safe to eat, but continue to engage in much more dangerous activity, for example, by driving their cars without buckling up.

Blaming the Victim

The reality of the human condition is that the body does wear down over time. If society becomes so health conscious that becoming sick is a sin (as already seems to be the case with AIDS), then the pendulum of holistic healing will have swung too far. Self-awareness is no doubt needed to assure good health and long life. At the same time, we must be careful not to blame the victim because some misfortunes in life are truly unavoidable. And not all dysfunction is a curable condition.[413] In this connection, Belch[414] decries the harsh mentality which presumes that sickness and other troubles can be attributed to an individual's moral deficiencies or lack of will power. In his view, we have permitted the pendulum to swing too far from the blind extreme of "It's always their fault" to the delusionary and self-destructive "It's always my fault." Both extremes veer equally far from truth. Belch argues that the current emphasis on personal responsibility has produced an unforgiving obsession with self-incrimination. The result often is a kind of indifference and unwillingness to accept the fact that some misfortunes will always persist, regardless of our best efforts to prevent or eliminate them. Moreover, living life to it fullest often means risking exposure to the potential for failure. Imperato and Mitchell[415] have put this in a somewhat broader context, noting that:

Life has always been full of risks, and some in fact have argued that a riskier life is a richer life; dancing on the edge of the abyss can be stimulating. For most people, however, most risks are genuinely unappealing most of the time. We may or may not be in greater peril than our ancestors—we don't die from smallpox but they didn't have to worry about The Bomb—but we are certainly more painfully aware of our vulnerability.

Deciphering a steady stream of alarming and sometimes ambiguous messages concerning threats to our well-being and survival is not an easy task. Part of the problem has to do with the "health hype" promulgated by the agents of the mass media, whereby minor health worries are often portrayed as major threats, and speculations about disease prevention are transformed into "proven" cures.[416] Taylor provides us with many examples of where the media has widely proclaimed very preliminary, weak, or even questionable findings as major medical breakthroughs. For example, in 1985, a team of French scientists announced at a press conference that the drug *cyclosporine* appeared to halt the growth of the AIDS virus. The announcement was based on observations of two AIDS patients treated for eight days. Ignoring the fact that no proper scientific study had been conducted, the media seized upon the announcement and made it a front-page story around the world. Unfortunately, one of the patients died within days. It turned out that cyclosporine was no miracle cure after all.

Scientists themselves sometimes purposely, often unwittingly, become collaborators in the spread of misinformation. The rules of science require that researchers first submit their work to peer review for evaluation and subsequent confirmation. However, in recent years we have seen many instances where investigators have ignored this important necessity and instead have moved quickly to public pronouncements concerning their often preliminary findings. Later, after careful scrutiny by other scientists has raised serious questions or doubts about the study, the investigator is forced to revise or retract the original pronouncement. Illustrative here are the experiments conducted by two scientists at the University of Utah, who proclaimed they had discovered a simple and easy way to trigger nuclear fusion at room temperature and pressure. Widespread scrutiny by the research community failed by and large to confirm their claims. Both men eventually suffered public humiliation, their reputations perhaps permanently damaged. A scientist announced that he and his colleagues had detected an apparent planet beyond the solar system. Six months later he reported, with obvious embarrassment, that the early analysis was flawed, and when corrected, "the planet just evaporated." The reasons why researchers engage in such premature dissemination of their findings are many. Often, however, such behavior reflects aspirations to "get there first," to secure funding, or to achieve personal recognition.[417]

Risk Minimalists and Avoidance Extremists

With increasing and widespread revelations about the hazards of living, many people will choose to join the ranks of either the risk minimalists, or the avoidance extremists. Somewhere in-between will be the moderate and perhaps majority group who consciously attempt to process the deluge of information in search of a rational and educated basis for making lifestyle choices. For these people all the knowledge they can get is welcomed and used. They recognize, however, that "health like any wealth can be pursued too ardently and hoarded too greedily.[418] Hence, they will pursue life giving a moderate amount of time and energy to avoiding unnecessary risks while ignoring other hazards they can do nothing about or they deem unworthy of further attention.

Excessive concern with health and longevity can in fact be counterproductive and lead to unreasonable expectations. Some believe we have already exceeded a balanced approach to quality living and in the process invited disappointment and failure. Ignatieff, for example, deplores the emergence of an almost maniacal pursuit of "the glow of physical well-being," insofar as it reflects an ideology of health which reduces the ideals of self-knowledge and self-mastery to unrealistic regimens of diet and exercise.[419] Within this context, health becomes a "dawn to dusk regimen" in which books on health replace those on philosophy as primary sources of enlightenment. He is especially critical of books which popularize psychoneuroimmunology, the science which focuses on the connections between psychological states of mind and the immune system. Many contend it offers an unrealistic promise—that one can prevent disease and improve health through the mastery of emotions. As we noted in an earlier chapter, the message of this new immunology of mind over matter is that through the exercise of our will we can control our fate. In his view, however, placing the burden of cure upon the individual can be "cruel to those unequal to the task." This may be especially true of the sick, who are apt to be accused of lacking adequate emotional strength and the will to resist. The result can be punitive: "If treatment fails you have no one to blame but yourself."

Ignatieff thinks we are discarding "a culture of endurance for a culture of complaint." In the past stoicism, which stressed the virtues of silent and heroic endurance, helped us to sustain a healthy acceptance of the limited influence of medicine on our destiny. However, with the conquest of so much illness stoic acquiescence of our biological fate is increasingly equated with weakness, passivity, fatalism, or a lack of personal responsibility—even moral failure. The idea that we control our destiny leads to an absurd belief in the injustice of death, that is, the conviction that death is unfair because it comes before we have managed to bring order to the story of our lives. This belief persists because we are convinced that "that we are the makers of our lives, when, in fact, chance and contingency and the dull determination of living all combined to push our lives into sequences we neither desire nor intend."

The refusal of each generation to accept the material and social limits that surrounded their lives has enabled mankind to live better, materially and morally, than those of the far past. But a culture that strongly stresses self-reliance, which no doubt has produced much good, is also susceptible to losing another good—a sense of fate. Many values of modernity conflict with another value: grace in the face of the fact of death. "To accept death," says Ignatieff, "is to accept much more than that we do not write the end of the story; it is also to appreciate that we don't write much of the beginning or the middle either."

Hence, he recommends "an ethic of ironic struggle," which means not too much struggle, not disproportionate struggle infused with mistaken moral meaning. His mentor is Montaigne who late in life was afflicted with a kidney stone at a time when the remedies of modern medicine were not available. Commenting on this experience, he demonstrates that acceptance of biological fate can at the same time be a form of self-mastery: "It is for my own good that I have the stone, it teaches me that buildings of my age must naturally suffer some leakage, that it is time for them to begin to grow loose and give way." Montaigne did not mean that we must go gently quiet into that good night. Rather, we should not rage against the dying of the light because all the health maintenance possible will not preclude our dying.

Unrealistic expectations can lead to a frantic pursuit of health, an insatiable desire for cures, and an inability to become reconciled to the limits of our transient presence on this earth. In Ignatieff's words: "Cultures that live by the values of self-realization and self-mastery are not especially good at dying, at submitting those experiences where freedom ends and biological fate begins." While a concern for our health and well-being is life-affirming and, therefore, a virtue, one needs to recognize that:

> ...within most virtues there lurks, waiting to slip its leash, a vice, in the form of excess. Any good, even the pursuit of longevity, can be pushed past its appropriate, its *natural* scope. The idealization of health is really a mere mate-

rialism, an obsession with bodily vitality and continuance…By all means jog. Just do not confuse maintenance with the conquest of mortality.[420]

Montaigne perhaps put it more succinctly when he wrote, "You do not die of being sick, you die of being alive."

16

The More Subtle Life Savers

Much of what has been discussed thus far deals with rather direct ways that people can improve their well-being through lifestyle changes—adhere to a good nutritional agenda, exercise and lose weight, don't smoke, avoid foolish risk-taking, be a defensive driver, get enough sleep, be positive in your approach to living, attempt to exert control over your life, eliminate life-threatening habits, and so on. Each of these actions can directly contribute to improving the length and quality of our lives. There are, however, other and less direct, often more subtle behaviors whose contributions to our well-being can easily be overlooked. Their importance should not be underestimated. They can in their own particular way, be life-saving.

Reading Can Be Life-Saving

Millions of Americans are illiterate. Millions of others can read, but choose not to. We now have an entire generation of people who spend more time each week watching television than practically any other activity. This is unfortunate because even a little reading can go a long way to ease the pain of living, reduce risky-living, or even prolong life. For example, one man noticed that over the past three years his breathing was getting progressively worse, despite thousands of dollars worth of medical tests to try and determine the cause. Then, one day while perusing through an issue of *Consumer Reports* he happened to read that **betoptic** was one of several glaucoma medications that can cause breathing problems, especially in asthmatics. He was using ***pilocarpine***, another glaucoma medicine. When he looked it up in a drug book, he found that it too can cause shortness of breath. He brought this information to his ophthalmologist, who then took him off the drug, and his breathing returned to normal.

Our popular press and scientific journals are filled with stories of people who neglected to read the instructions and other information printed on the inserts that accompany medications.[421] They subsequently found themselves the victims of dangerous drug interactions, sometimes with lethal consequences.[422] Most people, for example, probably don't know that there is a prescription drug that should never be taken with large amounts of caffeine. If a person were to drink a lot of coffee while taking *Inderal*, a drug used to regulate heart rhythm, it could soon raise their heartbeat to a dangerous rate. Most people, in fact, do not think of food, drink or over-the-counter products as interfering with drug therapy, but they can and they do. For instance, high doses of iron supplement can interfere with *Tetracycline*-type antibiotics by preventing them from being absorbed into the body. One could easily fill a book with such examples.

The more drugs one is taking, the more reason to read and become informed about possible interactions, due to the greater potential for harm. This is especially so among older persons, who generally tend to take more prescription drugs than younger persons. It has been estimated that 37 percent of those over 60 years of age are using five or more different prescription drugs, and that 19 percent are using seven or more. They have to be particularly careful, since certain drugs simply cannot be mixed and can lead to adverse reactions when taken in combination. One illustrative source of drug interaction in older people is the prescribed peptic ulcer drug *Tagamet*. If it is taken with *Theophylline*, a drug for breathing disorders such as asthma, it enhances the action of Theophylline and could induce a toxic reaction. The problem can be compounded by the fact that normal age-linked physical changes can make older persons more sensitive to side effects. Many physicians apparently fail to understand or sometimes forget that, given such susceptibility, older patients often need a lesser dosage of a given drug than those younger in order to achieve the desired effect.

Asking Questions Can Save Your Life

The author's parents were both born in Italy and migrated to the United States while relatively young. They soon met, married, and then proceeded to raise a large family of twelve children. Surviving in their new world was difficult and required considerable inner and outer strength as well as persistence. Many years later, when my father was in his eighties, I happen to ask him how as a young immigrant he managed to find his way through the myriad complexities of a foreign culture. His brief response: "When I didn't know, I asked." It turns out that asking questions can often help one avoid unnecessary trauma and survive. Often people avoid asking questions out of fear of being perceived as ignorant. Questioning, especially where it involved authority figures or experts, does call for a certain degree of confidence or assertiveness. For example, too often patients view their physicians as "drug givers" and themselves as "drug-receivers." This can result in a passive relationship in which they fail to query their physicians about the medications being prescribed and how to take them. They simply trot off to the pharmacy where another passive relationship may exist and again they hesitate to ask questions. Being inquisitive—asking and probing—in these and other life circumstances—can broaden one's knowledge and, more importantly, also prevent unnecessarily painful or dangerous outcomes.

Non-compliance Can Kill You

There is another side to this story. Non-compliance—the failure of patients to follow their physicians' preventive or therapeutic regimens—has been characterized as one of the most serious and costly epidemics in America today.[423] It is estimated that 125,000 people with treatable ailments die prematurely simply because they either failed to take prescribed medications properly, or to take them at all. This problem has been exacerbated in recent years with the growth in our elderly population who has chronic infirmities that require sustained treatment to avoid complications. Unfortunately, the elderly exhibit one of the highest rates of noncompliance. According to the National Council on Patient Information and Education, over 55 percent of elderly patients fail to take prescribed medication as directed. Related figures regarding the general population are rather startling:

> ...30 to 50 percent of all prescriptions dispensed by doctors are taken incorrectly by patients. One patient in five never even bothers to have the prescription filled. One in seven stops taking medication too soon, and nearly a third who do get their prescriptions the first time neglect to get refills ordered by their doctors...Taking a pill one or more times a day is hardly disruptive or time-consuming, yet half of all patients either neglect to do it or do it incorrectly.[424]

The problem, of course, is that many people are taking more than one pill during the day, and it can get very confusing trying to keep track of the different regimens.[425] Brody, whose report we have been drawing from, notes several of the most common reasons for noncompliance. For example, some patients stop taking their medication in order to avoid uncomfortable side effects. Such a decision is risky and can have life-threatening consequences, as in the case of illnesses like high blood pressure, which has few or no symptoms. Some people stop taking their medicine simply to see if it is still needed; again, a rather risky thing to do. Whatever the reason, making such decisions without consulting with the physician may be inviting unintended illness, disability, even death.

Attitudes Can Be Life-Saving

Throughout this book I have stressed the important role that attitudes play in survival. The cultivation of life-preserving attitudes can augment our well-being in a number of ways. One's philosophy of life not only influences the quality and vitality of daily living, but also contributes to longevity. Part of this philosophy embraces the notion of "paying attention" to each moment in life for its own sake and for the beauty it offers. In rereading and then evaluating the lessons she learned from the long, winding letters of her grandmother, who died at age 80, Cameron concluded that

> ...survival lies in sanity, and sanity lies in paying attention...the facts of life really have little to do with its quality. The quality of life is in proportion, always, to the capacity for delight. The capacity for delight is the gift of paying attention.[426]

Moreover, the act of paying attention brings with it the reward of healing.

Cameron also discovered that paying attention is an act of connection to all that is within our environment; that such connections give new meaning to life and enhance our ability to survive. She notes that it often takes some kind of pain to get people to pay attention to the discrete and precious moments of their existence. Pain forces us to re-evaluate our circumstances, to appreciate the value of right now, and to look forward to each moment of each day.

Those Who Lie with Dogs Get Fleas

Not infrequently, people engaging in behavior that threatens their health and longevity can be found associating with others who practice similar lifestyles. Hence, they are less apt to seriously criticize those lifestyles. Smokers more easily tolerate friends who smoke. The same can be said for those who are overweight, drink too much, and so on. The result can be what we might call *premature death by association*. The influence on us by others often takes place at an early age. For example, the National Center for Health Statistics conducted a survey of adolescents about their use of tobacco. Among their findings are two that are relevant to this discussion. First, teenagers were three times more likely to smoke if their parents and at least one older sibling smoked than if no one in the household smoked. Secondly, teenagers with no best friend of the same sex who smoked seldom smoked. However, about half of those with at least two best friends who smoked were smokers themselves.[427]

It is, of course, difficult to avoid family and friends who are engaging in risky behavior or unhealthy practices. Most of them will not be willing to change their behavior. The dilemma presents a real challenge. Nevertheless, to avoid illness or premature death, it may be necessary to develop new associations, ones that are more conducive to healthier lifestyles. Sometimes this might require moving to another environment where a person can more easily exercise different choices for living. For many, however, this option is beyond their reach. Ghetto neighborhoods dominated by a drug culture are a good example. Take the case of the heroin addicts who decides to reform and give up their life of drug abuse.

> ...Firm in this new resolve, they often return to their old neighborhood. Meeting old friends, they renew associations, go to a bar, or to a party. When the drugs emerge, it's too late for an effective choice...under those circumstances, the former addict cannot maintain his resolve, or has stacked the odds against success...Most treatment programs emphasize psychological hangups, and give lip service to relationships, but fail to provide alternatives for the addicts where they can begin to exert choices.[428]

Community treatment programs that assist addicts to relocate and to identify with reference groups that practice healthier lifestyles, and at the same time satisfy the addicts' need to belong, may give them a new lease on life. Instead of premature death by careless association, the result may be life preservation through caring association. This is not to underestimate the difficulties of curing addictive behaviors, of which there are many, but simply to recognize the potential inherent in reference groups, the strong influence such associations can have on life chances. "Support groups bring to bear on human problems the spiritual values of faith, hope, and charity. And whenever these virtues have been applied to the human condition, they have never failed to have a healing effect."[429]

The Life Sustaining Power of Hope

In an earlier chapter the relationship of cynicism to ill health and premature death was noted. The negative consequences flowing from feelings of hopelessness were similarly commented upon. For example, the loss of hope appears to be related to subsequent suicidal attempts. Thus, evidence is accumulating that persistence and feelings of hope can give people protective and survival advantages. One study, which compared two groups of people with paralysis from spinal cord injury, found that those reporting high levels of hope had less depression, greater mobility, more social contacts, and even more sexual intimacy than those expressing little hope.[430] Other studies of patients with serious diseases, such as congestive heart failure, have found that those who are more hopeful tend to maintain their involvement with life regardless of physical limitations. What is being suggested here is that "throwing in the towel," that is, giving up hope, can trigger negative outcomes and constrain life chances.

While the evidence may not be as clear cut as one would like, there are strong indications that intense determination or persistence, and hope, can have positive physiological effects. It has been found that such feelings actually can stimulate the spleen, thereby producing a rise in red blood cells and a corresponding increase in the number of cancer-fighting cells. There is even some suggestion that people that willfully summon positive attitudes or emotions to create changes in blood pressure, galvanic skin response and immune-system capability in order to combat illness and disease.[431]

Hopefulness, of course, bears some relationship to optimism, another life-extending attitude mentioned in previous pages. Some have even contended that this positive state of mind has a biological basis. Tiger, for example, in his book, *Optimism: The Biology of Hope*, asserts that optimism is a biological phenomena, which, like religion, "is rooted in human genes, which is why it keeps cropping up."[432] For Tiger, this basic attitude has played a key role in the evolution and perpetuation of humankind. Optimism, which connotes cheerfulness, confidence, and enthusiasm, is the opposite of pessimism, which implies cynicism and distrust. It sharply contrasts with despair, which connotes depression, melancholy, or resignation. It pays to be an optimist. Such people are better able to overcome depression, they tend to achieve more at school, work, or sports, they enjoy better health and, they may even live longer than pessimists. It appears that with practice this positive thinking and acting style can be learned.[433]

I am not suggesting a sort of mindless cheerfulness here. Rather, what is being called for is the development of what some have referred to as *flexible optimism*. This involves the ability to know when to adhere to a positive stance and when to give greater attention to the realism often associated with pessimism. A popular song sung by Kenny Rogers, *The Gambler*, captured this quite nicely in the line, "You've got to know when to hold 'um and know when to fold 'um." Shutting out *altogether* the warning signs sometimes signaled by a pessimistic perspective can lead to unnecessary risk-taking. "Life is a balancing act, and no one should be a slave to either mind-set."[434]

A Healthy Skepticism Doesn't Hurt Either

The Random House dictionary defines a skeptic as "a person who questions the validity or authenticity of something purporting to be factual." In searching for ways to avoid potential hazards to one's health, one might be wise to cultivate a healthy dose of skepticism. Earlier I discussed the notion that living is increasingly risky, at least if one were to believe the almost daily revelations about ordinary things that now presumably threaten our existence. There is little need to make life unnecessarily riskier by accepting dubious products claimed to be able to improve our health or cure our illnesses. The mass media is regularly used to promote the latest product designed to relieve symptoms or cure diseases. Given nationwide publicity, one might assume the product has been properly tested and the results validated. One could easily be wrong. Congressional hearings have revealed that the drug industry uses a wide variety of techniques to deceive and manipulate the mass media. Included among such practices were the passing off as independent experts physicians who are paid company spokespeople, toting as new breakthroughs drugs that actually offered little advantages over old formulas, and publicizing through press conferences and press releases unapproved and even untested drugs.[435] Many such testimonials, often done by well-known celebrities, or naive journalists, are seldom unbiased. Moreover, companies have been known to circumvent federal regulations regarding drug advertisements by promoting drugs under the guise of public education.

In an attempt to curb such practices, officials of the Federal Drug Administration began to assert it's authority over press releases, press conferences, video news releases, and other industry publicity tools. Federal law requires that promotionals must include both the positive *and* negative outcomes of prescription drugs. Moreover, the law prohibits the promotion of unapproved medications or unapproved uses of products already on the market. However, until specific formal guidelines are issued by federal agencies to cover the range of drug advertising and promotion, it remains questionable whether enforcement actions against specific companies will significantly alter prohibited practices. Given this uncertain situation, consumers would be wise to assert some protective skepticism, including a wariness toward the promotion of so-called "wonder drugs," especially if they are touted by celebrities. A questioning attitude regarding the scientific studies that form the basis for medical news reports is always in order. The report we have been citing offers several questions which should be asked, the answers to which can help persons judge a study and assist them in deciding whether to use the drug in question.[436]

Good Sleeping May Mean Healthier and Longer Living

There is some evidence that getting sufficient sleep—seven to eight hours for most of us—is essential to both the quality and the length of life. It has been noted that people who manage only six or less hours of sleep face a 70 percent chance of dying prematurely. Deficient sleep is associated with increased risks of heart trouble, digestive disease, female fertility problems, and serious or fatal accidents.

It has been estimated that 40 million Americans suffer from some form of *chronic* sleep disorder, and that half of them are afflicted by a condition called *apnea* (from the Greek word signifying not breathing). These people:

> actually stop breathing while asleep. As carbon dioxide builds up in the lungs, the brain senses something gone wrong and sounds its alarm, waking the person enough to activate the chest and diaphragm muscles. With a terrible snore, the lungs suck in fresh air. Sleep ends for the moment. This can happen 500 times a night—fracturing any peaceful, restorative slumber. During the day, the afflicted person, lacking a restful night, constantly dozes off.[437]

Apnea is experienced most often by people who are very overweight. However, it can and does affect slim persons as well. Researchers examining patients with moderate to severe sleep apnea found that those treated with continuous positive airway pressure (CPAP) devices had significant reductions in blood pressure during the day and night.[438] Another study of middle age women revealed that weight gain was linked to their amount of sleep The women who slept less were not only more threatened by weight gain but by obesity as well.[439] Taking sleeping pills generally gives only short-term relief. Eventually the body system develops a toleration for them and hence they lose their effect.

A variety of strategies have been developed which can be implemented to improving one' sleep pattern, for example, going to bed and getting up at the same time, and avoiding caffeine and other stimulants prior to going to bed.[440] Many such strategies have been found to be helpful to insomniacs—people who are unable to fall asleep easily—and nightshift workers, who must do their sleeping during the day.

The Therapeutic Benefits of Pet Ownership

Currently, Americans own over ninety million cats and seventy four million dogs and they often establish especial bonds with their animals. Nearly six million pet owners celebrate pet birthdays. It has been estimated that "the cost of caring for a medium-sized dog can go as high as $100.000, for those who make man's best friend their best friend."[441]

Evidence is accumulating to support the long-held suspicion that regular contact with animals can have specific and measurable positive effects on our mental and physical well-being. "The mere presence of animals can increase a sick person's chances of survival and has been shown to lower heart rate, calm disturbed children, and get incommunicative people to initiate conversations."[442] The mechanisms by which human-animal bonding influences health are little understood. Some believe that the benefits of animal companionship derive from the fact that, compared to human interaction, it is predictable and uncomplicated. "Animals are nonjudgmental, accepting and attentive; they don't talk back, criticize or give orders, they give people something to be responsible for and offer a non-threatening outlet for physical contact."[443] Others suggest that the opportunities for caring nurturance provided by the presence of an animal can lead to healing outcomes. For example, the experience of helping a wounded or ill pet to recuperate may enhance a person's feeling of worthiness and perhaps even their will to live.

Animals can also positively affect our physical well-being. "Heart rate, for example, is lower when people sit quietly or read aloud in the presence of a friendly animal, than when doing so alone."[444] There is some evidence of higher survival rates among heart surgery patients with pets in their homes than among those with none. Moreover, elderly pet owners apparently make fewer visits to physicians than those without animal companionship. This suggests that such having a pet somehow helps mitigate the negative consequences of prolonged loneliness. Perhaps it provides the comfort and companionship that the elderly might otherwise seek from visits to their doctors. It is not unknown for people to talk to their pets. Perhaps what all this illustrates, in the broadest sense, is that for many people a little bit of love can go a long way.

You Can Live Longer

The title of a recent article on staying alive was "Can You Live Longer?"[445] It answers the question in the affirmative, and suggests that people can maximize their longevity by following many of the risk-reduction strategies discussed in this book, for example, eating a well-balanced, low-fat, high-carbohydrate diet, exercising regularly, refraining from smoking and alcohol abuse, and avoiding obesity.[446] These are things we can do to enhance both the quality and quantity of life. There are others.

Simplicity and Moderation. No one would disagree that the world and our daily existence has become increasingly complex with each passing decade. That complexity brings with it many benefits as well as many drawbacks, for example, widespread stress. For contemporary men and women to maximize their survival potential, strategies must be followed which minimize those drawbacks. This involves what was described in an earlier chapter as *self-watching*, a concept which embraces self-awareness, self-responsibility, self-empowerment, and self-appreciation. It means consciously avoiding those behaviors which are deleterious to your health, and at the same time engaging in behaviors which contribute to your well-being.

One key to achieving wellness is to simplify your life—admittedly not always an easy thing to do. But this can be done in numerous little ways. There is little question that the longer one lives, the more complex life becomes. To keep that complexity from diminishing life chances requires "unburdening yourself of all that prevents the natural state of basic healthiness from being present."[447] This means, among other things, taking control of your life by getting rid of a great deal of unnecessary baggage, for example, overinvolvements and overcommitments, in order to lead a healthier and more satisfying existence. It means getting rid of the array of trivia that can aggravate and provoke us into wasting time and energy; that is, learning to distinguish between the details of life that are worth worrying about and those that are not.[448] In an earlier chapter we referred to this as learning to shield yourself from the little hassles of daily living. Our culture has many sayings which reflect this philosophic pragmatism. For example, the idea that getting bogged down in details prevent us from "being able to separate the forest from the trees." Those who strive too hard for perfectionism often spend so much time and energy struggling over the minute details that they fail to achieve the larger objectives. As John Updike once noted in his book *Odd Jobs*: "Perfectionism is the enemy of creation, as extreme self-solicitude is the enemy of well-being."

In sum, keeping one's eye on the bigger picture and paying attention to details within reasonable limits can contribute to our well-being. And altering or avoiding the myriad of unnecessary yet emotionally draining irritations of life, especially in the area of human interaction, is essential. This means, as we noted earlier, withdrawing from those relationships which diminish and demean us, and shifting to others which provide dependable affection and care.

Another key to staying alive is to adhere to the path of moderation. Many people seem to abandon rational restraint in favor of overindulgence. The results can be risky and life-threatening. Conniff illustrates this with the story of Luigi Cornaro, a sixteenth century Paduan, who:

> …was such a profligate youth that by the time he was 40, he found his constitution "utterly ruined by a disorderly way of life and by frequent overindulgences in sensual pleasure." Told to reform, he entered upon the *vita sobria*, a life of moderation in all things. He restricted himself in particular to just twelve ounces of food daily and lived in robust health until he was 98.[449]

Conniff not only used Cornaro to illustrate the value of moderation, but also to indicate the value of undernutrition—as distinguished from malnutrition. He observes that some modern scientific experiments with animals whose diet was restricted after they became adults achieved a 30 percent increase in maximum life span. "The crucial refinement seems to have been moderation." In these experiments, underfeeding not only delayed death, it also delayed aging in the test animals. The implications for humans here are rather clear and confirm what we have always intuitively known, namely, that a life of excess carries with it the potential for illness and early demise.

17

The Politics of Survival

Individual and Community Initiatives

I have noted the difficulty of protecting our well-being in the face of inexact and often contradictory information regarding the risks associated with facets of our lifestyles. I have also commented on the role that political ideology plays in regulating threats to our welfare imposed by business and industry. It is not unusual for politicians and scientists to sharply disagree over questions of risk. Nor is it unusual to find each using the *same* studies of the health risks surrounding a particular issue to support their position. This is due in part to the imprecision which currently characterizes the fledgling science of risk analysis or assessment.[450] That inexactitude opens the door for conflicting interpretations. Consequently: "Instead of being used to decrease the biggest risks to life, risk analysis frequently becomes a weapon used in the wars between regulators and their opponents."[451]

Illustrative here is a confrontation between politicians, industry, and scientists concerning the harmful effects of cadmium dust and fumes. In this case the Occupational Safety and Health Administration was considering imposing more stringent exposure rules in order to better protect the health of the workers. This proposal, of course, was opposed by the cadmium industry. It subsequently enlisted the aid of federal lawmakers who represented districts with cadmium companies, a White House agency that reviews regulatory proposals, certain other governmental agencies and departments, and then Vice-President Dan Quayle's Council on Competitiveness.

All agreed that exposure to high doses of cadmium, a toxic industrial metal used to coat metals and to make batteries and pigments, can damage kidneys and possibly cause lung cancer. They vehemently disagreed, however, on how dangerous cadmium might be at lower levels of exposure. Industry representatives utilized critics of risk analysis to challenge the research findings upon which the OSHA proposal was based. Eventually the parties concerned, under pressure of a court order, pursued a politically expedient compromise, but leaving the issue as to what level of cadmium is dangerous to worker health unresolved.

What Is Carcinogenic-Anyway?

At various points we have noted the weekly or monthly pronouncements that appear in the media concerning the latest, sometimes frightening carcinogenic discovery. Often these pronouncements emanated from verdicts issued by the National Toxicology Program, an entity responsible for testing substances for possible cancer-causing properties. Its conclusions serve as the basis for far-reaching regulatory actions by other government agencies charged with overseeing the health and safety of citizens, such as the Environmental Protection Agency, the Food and Drug Administration, the Occupational Safety and Health Administration, the Agriculture Department, the Consumer and Product Safety Commission, as well as many state and local regulatory bodies.

Under this program, substances are tested in animals at what is known as the *maximum tolerated dose*, that is, the highest amount compatible with their survival, in order to encourage the appearance of cancer. Going beyond such levels would in all likelihood kill the test animals. Several assumptions underlie this approach, namely that:

1. the rates at which a substance is absorbed, distributed and eliminated by the body are the same regardless of the dose;

2. when maximum tolerated doses produce cancer in animals, the same cancers will be produced in proportion to smaller doses, no matter how small;

3. the rate at which the body repairs toxic genetic damage is unaffected by the dose of toxic substance absorbed;

4. the likelihood of developing cancers is not influenced by the age of the animals;

5. the maximum tolerated dose can be higher—hundreds or thousands of times higher—than likely human doses.[452]

A report was issued by the Program's Board of Scientific Counselors which challenged the validity of these assumptions, questioning whether they are scientifically tenable.

If the conclusions of the report are upheld, the implication would be that many substances previously tested by the Toxicology Program may have been improperly classified as carcinogenic. If so, changes will be needed regarding the way the Program tests substances in animals and evaluates the results in terms of possible human risk. This may mean that hundreds of substances listed in the past as carcinogenic will have to be re-evaluated and reclassified according to the new criteria. As a result, many may no longer be classified as carcinogens. Hence, a continuance of the regulations governing their use would be difficult to justify.

Community Response: An Emergent Survival Strategy

In an earlier discussion of *contaminated communities*, the stressful process experienced by those attempting to cope with the immediate and long-term threats from toxic exposure, was noted. It was observed that frequently such incidents lead to distrust and conflict between government and industry representatives, charged with resolving such crises, and the exposed citizens. Frustrated by such encounters, people in the affected neighborhoods or communities have increasingly found themselves forced to organize at the grass roots level in order to gain adequate leverage in their efforts to achieve a solution to the problem. As more homes and communities experienced toxic exposure, and as the view that such widespread incidents posed an insidious social problem gained broader awareness, an organized social movement on the part of the people affected emerged. It encourages active, citizen based initiatives as a strategy in getting their concerns adequately represented in dealing with the life-threatening conditions of toxic exposure and environmental pollution. An organized, grass roots response can serve as a "therapeutic social system" that helps "compensate for the stress of disasters by sharing information, warmth, and help; providing a means for rapid consensus about actions necessary to meet collective needs; and engendering a high degree of motivation among victims to work for common purposes."[453]

Researchers have identified several key outcomes from the grass roots response to technological disasters or risks posed by toxic exposure. Among these outcomes are *social support*, which provides the citizens with reassurance and strength when encountering a collective predicament; *shared information*, made possible as neighborhood communication lines are opened to deal with the impending threat, which people feel they can believe and trust; and *power*, allowing individuals and families to overcome their initial sense of helplessness, and to take collective actions on issues they would hesitate to tackle alone. In the latter connection, grass roots organizations, or what some refer to as "reactive community groups," will often utilize experts to help them address the complex issues resulting from toxic exposure. Not only can experts also help them understand the significance of new developments or plot strategy, but they also can take on adversaries directly. "Through their collective activities and ability to attract resources, community organizations provide a means of attaining the power needed to address the complex issues resulting from toxic exposure."[454]

An example of how citizens come to recognize and then deal with the problem of toxic waste contamination was provided by the community of Woburn, Massachusetts.[455] Residents of this working-class and lower-middle-class town, located a dozen miles north of Boston, traced groundwater contamination by known carcinogens to certain local industries. They then sought to link exposure to this water to an elevated frequency of leukemia in children. A prolonged confrontation ensued, during which they fought against the corporations involved, and at the same time grappled with local, state, and federal officials and scientists. Eventually, citizen initiatives, by way of organized community action, won a court battle and out-of-court financial settlements as partial compensation for the affected families. The researchers who studied this case analyzed how local community members became activists who mobilized other citizens behind the cause, the reactions of various constituencies in the town, and the resistant roles played by state and federal health and environmental agencies. They also examined the inherently oppositional vested interest of the corporations that owned the factories, as well as the range of health effects, psychological stress, social disruptions, and pain experienced by the affected families and other community members.

Popular Epidemiology. The medical sociologist and psychiatrist who conducted a detailed analysis of this particular case employed the concept of *popular epidemiology*, suggesting it as a model which can be emulated by other communities. Unlike traditional epidemiology, that focuses on the distribution of illness or disease and their causes, popular epidemiology:

> is the process by which laypersons gather scientific data and other information and direct and marshal the knowledge and resources of experts to understand the epidemiology of disease...popular epidemiology is more than a matter of public participation in traditional epidemiology. Popular epidemiology goes further in emphasizing social structural factors as part of the causative chain of disease, in involving social movements, in utilizing political and judicial remedies, and in challenging basic assumptions of traditional epidemiology, risk assessment, and public health regulation.[456]

This is a process, then, whereby lay citizens conduct the painstaking data collection themselves, and enlist the assistance of sympathetic scientists who can design valid research methods for small populations and amateur researchers. For example, in the Woburn case, the citizens' activist organization enlisted expert help from several biostatisticians. They eventually made a convincing case that a leukemia "cluster" existed, with rates four times the expected levels.

Popular epidemiology is one example of how to promote meaningful public participation in scientific work relating to toxic problems. Proponents of this approach are sympathetic to the interests of toxic waste victims, whose claims are often subverted by influential corporate, political, and even scientific establishments. Hence, they advocate policies to enhance public knowledge of environmental problems, and which force corporations to become legally and morally more responsible for the health problems they create.[457] They also encourage policies which make government agencies more responsive to the interest of lay community members faced with severe environmental problems. In their efforts to correct problems that have not been resolved by the established corporate, political, and scientific communities, environmental health activists have proven to be effective agents of change. There is evidence that they "have significantly advanced public health and safety by pointing out otherwise unidentified problems and showing how to approach them, by organizing to abolish the conditions that give rise to them, and by educating citizens, public agencies, health care providers, officials, and institutions."[458]

Raising Our Risk-Consciousness

Despite the various difficulties which characterize contemporary risk analysis and assessment,[459] and the obstacles to correcting the man-made hazards which confront us, we certainly must—and we can—raise our risk-consciousness, and follow strategies that reduce our vulnerability to personal and societal life-threatening environments. By doing so, we will strengthen our survival capability. These strategies, which involve conscious activity designed to minimize if not to avoid exposure to fatal illnesses and encounters, comprise those elements of *death education* that contribute to the art of living. Rene Dubois noted many years ago that: "To ward off disease or recover health, men as a rule find it easier to depend on the healers than to attempt the more difficult task of living wisely." Reducing our dependence on the healers will require a shift away from those attitudes and lifestyles which diminish the quality and length of our existence. To achieve our healthiest potential, we will have to more consciously assess the chances we take and assume the liability for the outcomes. One need not shirk from actively engaging life, but that engagement should be tempered by a more rational approach to living, or what some have called *preventive living*. It involves a philosophy that is geared to encouraging behavior that preserves health. This is what I think DuBois meant about living wisely. It is a philosophy embraced by what has come to be known as the *wellness movement*. This rapidly growing movement, broadly speaking, promotes a concept of wellness as "a conscious and deliberate approach to an advanced state of physical and psychological/spiritual health," and as "a dynamic or ever-changing, fluctuating state of being."[460] In more concrete terms, the proponents of this movement emphasize a conscious commitment to wellness lifestyles by adhering to healthy life habits.

In the early chapters I discussed the A, B, and C personality types in relation to predispositions to illness. Implied throughout this book has been a call for the Type H (Health) personality. These are people whose lifestyles are commensurate with quality living.[461] They have taken the fitness *revolution* seriously, and have changed their habits with respect to self-care. Among other things, they reguarly exercise, which improves self-esteem and helps them to adapt to stress; they openly express emotions; they have learned how and when to relax; they consciously follow a proper diet; and they maintain a positive outlook on life. They believe that to stay younger for longer they must remain physically and mentally active, an attitude summarized by the now well known expression "use it or lose it." These are psychologically and socially mature people who have recognized their unhealthy patterns of thinking and acting and then deliberately set out to replace them with more life-sustaining patterns.[462]

Overcoming Our Comfort Zones

Embarking on such a program and remaining committed to its continuation are not easy. It requires overcoming a natural and often strong resistance to change in order to achieve new goals. This means breaking free from well entrenched negative habits and routines which we recognize as unhealthy but nevertheless retain because we have become altogether too comfortable with them. In more general terms, it means transcending the boundaries of our personal *comfort zones* and testing our ability to change.[463] This can be somewhat frightening or intimidating, since one doesn't know whether one will succeed or fail. The experience is not unlike those felt by athletes who, aware of the possibility of failure, nevertheless constantly seek to test the limits of their abilities in order to achieve new goals. Such people would be unable to set new records unless they were willing to take a chance—to "go for the gold," so to speak. In a somewhat related fashion, overcoming habitualized patterns of living also requires overcoming a fear of failure, a sustained effort to make the changes desired, and it involves some degree of risk. There is a cautionary note, however, with regard to moving beyond our comfort zones.

> You want and need to take risks, but not ones that are too big…A risk that's too great puts us into overwhelm. If every risk puts you into overwhelm, your life is devoted to running scared, and that is not a way to live. You've got to find a happy medium.[464]

In short, biting off more than you can chew can prevent your accomplishing your goal.[465]

Within the above context, living on the middle ground, practicing a life of moderation if you will, while at the same time exposing yourself to calculated forms of risk-taking, becomes a worthy goal. Indeed, civilization itself would not have progressed if all people avoided involvements whose outcomes were not known in advance. It's been suggested that if our ancestors had insisted on a maximum of certainty in their lives, they might never have emerged from the caves. "It was the search for the good things in life while risking the bad that set people on the road to civilization."[466] And with the advent of civilization many hazards of the world have become more manageable. Disease and life-shortening events are increasingly understood and brought under control through innovative technologies. However, these same changes in technology often brought with them new kinds of risks. Fortunately a "spirit of prudence" has evolved to counterbalance the new "spirit of boldness," created by harnessing new threats in our living environments.

The essential balance between boldness and prudence has wavered from time to time, sometimes with destructive consequences, such as war and social stagnation. This historical process continues today, both at the societal and individual levels. The process always takes place within an ever-present context of uncertainty, which for some is a constant source of anxiety and tension over what the future portends. The best strategy to allay such apprehensions, and to deal effectively with prospective perils "is to isolate the ones you can do something about, and do something about them—and stop worrying about the rest."[467] From experience people learn how to make decisions in their own lives, balancing the costs versus the rewards to make intelligent choices. Some might try to insulate themselves from the unpredictability of events and circumstances, but they cannot succeed for very long. Why? Because, "life itself is uncertain—we cannot depend on its continuance. The only real certainty for any of us is death."[468]

A realistic and at the same time more optimistic approach to living, and one that is apt to contribute to both the quality and longevity of our earthly existence is essential to survival. The essence of that approach is captured in some remarks by Gerald W. Paul, writing in an issue of *The Elks*. Its message perhaps constitutes an appropriate philosophy with which to conclude:

> Our lives are somewhat fixed by fate, partly in the cards. The power of positive thinking will not turn paraplegics into quarterbacks or the blind into astronomers. But while a leopard can't change its spots, it can change its habits. Genes may make us susceptible to diabetes, but we can reduce the risk by avoiding obesity. Nature may play a role in lung cancer, but we can quit smoking. Inheritance may include a bad heart, but appropriate exercise may be a winning card. For in life, as in poker, you don't need a royal flush to be a winner. Sometimes a pair of deuces—a weak hand played well—is plenty.

Endnotes

Notes to the Preface

1. Felix M. Berardo, "Survivorship: The Other Side of Death and Dying," <u>Death Studies</u>, Vol. 9, No. 1, 1985, pp. 1-93.

2. Melvin Konner, Why the Reckless Survive . . . and Other Secrets of Human Nature, New York: Viking, p. vii.

3. Research on disasters, such as that of Hurricane Katrina, seeks to understand "that disasters are the result of a complex relationships between a potentially damaging event and the general vulnerability of a society, its economy, and the environment. And to reduce the risk of disasters happening in the future is essential that we find out how vulnerable we are now." Joern Birkmann, "Danger need not spell disaster But how vulnerable are we?" United Nations University Research Brief, Number 1, 2005, p. 1.

Notes to the Introduction

4. Wayne King, "Survivalists Are Stocking Up to Prepare For Doomsday," <u>Gainesville Sun</u>, January 25, 1981, p. 16E.

5. Peter Arnett, "Survival of the Fittest Is Their Only Concern," <u>Gainesville Sun</u>, March 2, 1981, p. 2D.

6. Lynn Langway, et al., "The Doomsday Boom," <u>Newsweek</u>, August 11, 1980, p. 56.

7. D. Pearson and S. Shaw, <u>Life Extension</u>, New York: Warner, 1982.

8. D. Pearson and S. Shaw, <u>The Life Extension Companion</u>, New York: Warner, 1984.

9.   David Stipp, "Studies Showing Benefits of Antioxidants Prove Potent Tonic for Sales of Vitamin E," The Wall Street Journal, April 13, 1993, pp. B1 and B6.

10. Roy L. Walford, Maximum Life Span, New York: Norton, 1983.

11. "Can You Live Longer? What Works and What Doesn't," Consumer Reports, January, 1992, pp. 7-15.

12. Daniel Callahan, Setting Limits: Medical Goals in an Aging Society, New York: Simon and Schuman, 1987.

13. Robert L. Barry and Gerard V. Bradley (Editors), Set No Limits, A Rebuttal to Daniel Callahan's Proposal to Limit Health Care for the Elderly, Baltimore, MD: University of Illinois Press, 1992.

14. "Can You Live Longer?" Consumer Reports, January, 1992, pp. 7-15.

15. Kathleen Stein, "Some of Us May Never Die," Omni, October, 1978.

16. Robert G. Evans, Morris L. Barer, and Theodore R. Marmor (Editors), Why Are Some People Healthy and Others Not?, New York: Aldine De Gruyter, 1994, p. ix.

17. Malcolm Boyd, "What Makes A Survivor?" Modern Maturity, April-May, 1994, p. 72.

18. Michael A. Simpson, The Fear of Death, Englewood Cliffs, New Jersey: Prentice-Hall, 1979.

19. Felix M. Berardo (Editor), "Survivorship: The Other Side of Death and Dying." A Special Issue of Death Studies, Vol. 9, 1985, pp. 1-75.

20. Alvin R. Tarlov, "The Spectrum of Health: Matching Medical Education to Medical Realities," in Russell C. Maulitz (Editor) Unnatural Causes: The Three Leading Killer Diseases in America, New Brunswick, NJ: Rutgers University Press, 1989, p. 189.

21. Ibid, p. 187.

22. Epidemiology has been formally defined as the "study of the distribution and determinants of health-related states or events in specified populations, and the application of this study to control of health problems." Or, in the words of one epidemiologist, it is "the study of our collective health" (Rockett, 1994, p. 2).

23. Ian R.H. Rockett, "Population and Health: An Introduction to Epidemiology," <u>Population Bulletin</u>, Vol. 49, No. 3, November, 1994, p. 12.

24. Michael J. Apter, <u>The Dangerous Edge: The Psychology of Excitement</u>, New York: The Free Press, 1992.

25. H. Feifel, "The Meaning of Death in American Society: Implications for Education," in B.R. Green and D.P. Irish (Editors), <u>Death Education: Preparation for Living</u>, Cambridge, MA: Schenkan, 1971.

26. Felix M. Berardo, "Introduction," <u>Death Studies</u>, Vol. 9, 1985, pp. 1-4.

27. The emphasis on longevity does not mean I favor it over the quality of life. The fullness of life, most would agree, is not related to years alone but also to the caliber of our existence.

Notes to Chapter 1

28. Felix M. Berardo, "The Role of Habits, Attitudes, and Risk Taking," <u>Death Studies</u>. Vol. 10 (1985), pp. 391-409.

29. J.E. Knott, "Death Education For All," in H. Wass (Editor), <u>Dying: Facing the Facts</u>, New York: Hemisphere, 1979.

30. M. Renaud, "The Future: Hygeia versus Panakeia?" in Robert G. Evans, Morris L. Barer, and Theodore R. Marmor (Editors) <u>Why Are Some People Healthy and Others Not?</u>, New York: Aldine De Gruyter, 1994, p. 320.

31. A.M. Brandt, "The Cigarette, Risk, and American Culture," <u>Daedalus</u>, (FAll, 1990), pp. 155-176.

32. Ralph Keyes, <u>Chancing It: Why We Take Risks</u>, Boston, MA: Little, Brown, 1985, pp. 9-11.

33. Even a perusal of the scientific journal <u>Risk Analysis</u> will quickly give readers some idea of the wide ranging and highly technical treatment given this topic by professional researchers.

34. William W. Lowrance, <u>Of Acceptable Risk: Science and the Determination of Safety</u>, Los Altos, CA: William Kaufmann, 1976.

35. P.J. Imperarto and G. Mitchell, <u>Acceptable Risks</u>, New York: Viking, 1985.

36. J. Urquhart and K. Heilmann, <u>Risk Watch</u>. New York: Facts on File, 1985.

37. Eleanor Singer and Phylllis M. Endreny, <u>Reporting ON Risk: How the Mass Media Portrays Accidents, Diseases, Disasters, and Other Hazards</u>, New York: Russell Sage Foundation, 1993.

38. However, the theory behind the scale is not quite this simple because it takes into account only the risk of death for people included in a special cohort—those who smoke. Urquhart and Heilmann denote this cohort at risk in any given activity as a "unicohort," and they derive their scale from this group (p.46). While the unicohort for smoking risks consists of just smokers, the unicohort for being struck by lightening encompasses every human being.

39. William Beery, et al., <u>Health Risk Appraisal: Methods and Programs, with Annotated Bibliography</u>, Washington, D.C.: National Center for Health Services Research and Health Care Technology Assessment, June, 1986.

40. Steven Findlay, "Healthy Living by the Numbers," <u>U.S. News & World Report</u>, April 11, 1988, p. 64.

41. Singer and Endreny, 1993, p. 2.

42. Bill Bryson, "Life's Little Gambles," <u>The Saturday Evening Post, September, 1988.</u>

43. Health-risk appraisal programs have become commercially attractive. Numerous companies now market computerized profiles directly to consumers. Many employers offer them for a nominal fee or sometimes free as part of the employment health-care package.

44. "None of an Employer's Business," <u>New York Times</u>, July 7, 1991.

45. Barbara Kantrowitz, et al., "The Pregnancy Police," <u>Newsweek</u>, April 29, 1991, pp. 52-53.

46. "Risk-Takers Rebel Against Helplessness," <u>St. Petersburg Times</u>, August 2, 1982, p. 30.

47. J. Carey, et al., "New Wave Mountain Men," <u>Newsweek</u>, October 1, 1984, pp. 82-83.

48. "Risk-Takers Rebel Against Helplessness," <u>St. Petersburg Times</u>, August 2, 1982, p. 30.

49. John Underwood, "It's Pretty, It's Trendy, but Skiing Is Also Much Too Dangerous," <u>New York Times</u>, February 26, 1995, p. 23.

50. Tom Lyons, "Student Drinks Himself to Death," <u>The Gainesville Sun</u>, November 6, 1991, pp. 1 and 4A.

51. William Celis 3d, "Fewer on Campuses Drink but Deadly Abuses Endure," <u>The New York Times</u>, December 31, 1991, pp. A1 and A14.

52. R. Jessor, "Psychological Correlates of Marijuana Use and Problem Drinking in a National Sample," <u>American Journal of Public Health</u>, Vol. 70 (1980), pp. 604-614.

53. C. Lewis and M.A. Lewis, "Peer Pressure and Risk Taking Behaviors in Children," <u>American Journal of Public Health</u>, Vol. 74, 1984, pp. 580-584.

54. L.A. DeSpelder and A.E. Strickland, <u>The Last Dance: Encountering Death and Dying</u>, Palo Alto, CA: Mayfield, 1983, p. 311.

55. Bill Richards, "Alaska's Denali Attracts the Hardy and the Foolhardy," <u>Wall Street Journal</u>, June 27, 1994, p. B1.

56. "Dealing With Danger," <u>The Royal Bank Newsletter</u>, Vol. 61, July, 1980, p. 6.

57. "Making Up Our Minds," The Royal Bank Newsletter, Vol. 68, September/October, 1987, p. 2.

58. Kinney Bennett, "How Lucky People Get That Way," Reader's Digest, March, 1991, pp. 128-132.

59. "Dealing With Danger," The Royal Bank Newsletter, July, 1980.

60. Urquhart and Heilmann, Risk Watch, p. xiii.

61. "Living With Uncertainty," The Royal Bank Newsletter, Vol. 68, March/April, 1987, p. 1.

62. Ibid. p. 1.

Notes to Chapter 2

63. Jessica Field Cohen," Male Roles in Mid-Life," The Family Coordinator, Vol. 28, October, 1979, pp. 465-471.

64. F.M. Berardo, Social Adaptation to Widowhood Among a Rural-Urban Aged Population, Washington Agricultural Experiment Station, Technical Bulletin 689, Pullman: Washington State University, 1967.

65. Redford B. Williams, The Trusting Heart: Great News About Type A Behavior, New York: Random House, 1989.

66. John Carey with Mary Bruno, "Why Cynicism Can Be Fatal," Newsweek, September 10, 1984, p. 68.

67. Norman Cousins, "Hope Can Make You Well," Parade Magazine, October 29, 1989, pp. 12-13.

68. Ibid.

69. "Funny You Should Ask," Health Scene, Winter, 1990, p. 3.

70. Ibid.

71. Cousins own illness and recovery experience convinced him that emotions can play a profound part in bringing on disease and in helping to combat it. Prior to his death in 1991 he had published two volumes on the subject.

Anatomy of an Illness, and later *The Healing Heart: Antidotes to Panic and Helplessness.*

72. Norman Cousins, "What you Believe and Feel Can Have an Effect on Your Health," U.S. News & World Report, January 23, 1984, pp. 61-62.

73. More stringent regulations governing research involving human subjects no longer permit "placebo surgery."

74. Peter E.S. Freund and Meredith B. McGuire, Health, Illness, and the Social Body: A Critical Sociology, Englewood Cliffs, New Jersey: Prentice Hall, 1991, p. 75-80.

75. Barron H. Lerner, "An old idea: What Ails the Body is Rooted in the Mind." New York Times, May 2, 2006.

76. Anees A. Sheikh, "Pictures of Health," Omni, February, 1989, pp. 105-112.

77. Time Magazine, June 24, 1985.

78. B.S. Seigel, Love, Medicine, and Miracles: Lessons Learned About Self-Healing From A Surgeons's Experience With Exceptional Patients, New York: Harper & Row, 1988.

79. M. Ignatieff, "Modern Dying," The New Republic, December 26, 1988, pp. 28-33.

80. Sontag, Susan, Illness as Metaphor, New York: Farrar Strauss and Giroux, 1978.

81. Bill Moyers, Healing And The Mind, New York: Doubleday, 1993.

82. David P. Phillips and Kenneth A. Feldman, "A Dip In Deaths Before Ceremonial Occasions: Some New Relationships Between Social Integration and Mortality," American Sociological Review, Vol. 38 December, 1973, pp. 678-696.

83. Myron Boor, "Effects of United States Presidential Elections on Suicide and Other Causes of Death," American Sociological Review, Vol. 46 (1981), pp. 616-618. However, these findings have been challenged by

others. For a discussion of the issues, see: Myron Boor and Jerome A. Flem-ing, "Presidential Election Effects on Suicide and Mortality Levels Are Independent of Unemployment Rates," <u>American Sociological Review</u>, Vol. 49 October, 1984, pp. 706-709.

84.   Interestingly, the investigators also found that famous groups of people experience a larger than expected death-dip as well as a greater death-peak than the non-famous.

85.   Farley found some gender differences among financial risk takers. For example, compared to female financial adventurers, men are more apt to drink hard liquor, go to the racetrack, steal, or own guns. These differences may simply reflect the influence of sex role definitions. The men also felt that they were more prone to take physical risks and to have greater control over their lives than their female counterparts.

86.   Cindy Skrzycki, et al., "Risk Takers," <u>U.S. News & World Report</u>, January 26, 1987, pp. 60-67.

87.   The previous list draws heavily from Skrzycki. See References.

88.   Skrzycki, 1987, p. 62

89.   J.A. Thornson and Powell, "Factor Structure of a Lethal Behavior Scale," <u>Psychology Reports</u>, Vol. 61, 1987, pp. 807-810.

90.   G. Keinen, et al., "Measurement of Risk Takers' Personality," <u>Psychology Reports</u>, Vol. 55, 1984, pp. 163-167.

91.   J.W. Atkinson, "Motivational Determinants of Risk Taking Behavior," <u>Psychology Review</u>, Vol. 64, 1957, pp. 358-361.

92.   Alvin P. Sanoff, "The Legacy of Our Genes," <u>U.S. News & World Report</u>, January 14, 1991, p. 53. Report of an interview with Melvin Konner, author of <u>Why the Reckless Survive . . . And Other Secrets of Human Nature</u>, Viking Press, 1991.

93.   A. Roy, et al., "Pathological Gambling,: <u>Archives of General Psychiatry</u>, April, 1988, pp. 369-373.

94. Sharon Begley with Daniel Glick and Larry Wilson, "Not in the Stars, But in Our Genes," <u>Newsweek</u>, October 21, 1991, pp. 56-57.

Notes to Chapter 3

95. John B. Baldwin, "Habit, Emotion, And Self-Conscious Action," <u>Sociological Perspectives</u>, Vol. 31, No. 1, January, 1988, pp. 35-58.

96. U.S. Department of Health and Human Services, <u>Healthy People 2000: National Health Promotion and Disease Prevention Objectives</u>, Washington, D.C.: U.S. government Printing Office, 1991.

97. Lee Goldman and E. Francis Cook, "The Decline in Ischemic Heart Disease Mortality Rates," <u>Annals of Internal Medicine</u>, Vol. 101, 1984, pp. 825-836.

98. Jane E. Brody, "7 Deadly Sins of Living Linked To Illness as Well as Mortality," <u>The New York Times</u>, May 12, 1993, p. B6.

99. Elliot Carlson, "Join the Wellness Revolution," <u>Modern Maturity</u>, (June-July, 1986), pp. 39, 89, 92-98.

100. Some experts disagree with this conclusion, arguing that such studies fail to take into account so-called "robust survivors"—people who apparently disregard many of the risk factors discussed in this book, and yet still survive. They contend that many people reach later age without succumbing to such factors because they simply are not susceptible to them. However, since we have no way of knowing whether we are one of these robust types, prudence would lead us to adhere to a healthier regimen.

101. Lester Breslow and Norman Breslow, Lester Breslow and Norman Breslow, <u>Preventive Medicine</u>, 1993.

102. Jane E. Brody, "7 Deadly Sins of Living Linked to Illness as well as Mortality," The New Yor Times, May 12 1993.

103. Fred Cutter, <u>Coming to Terms With Death</u>, Chicago: Nelson-Hall, 1974, p. 81.

104. Not all habitual activities, of course, are of a voluntary nature. Through repetition and association with certain stimuli habitual responses can become automatic and eventually compulsive or involuntary.

105. "The Cancer Scourge: Early Detection Can Save Thousands of Lives," Newsweek, June 9, 1986, p. 69.

106. "The Dark Side of the Sun," Newsweek, June 9, 1986, p. 60.

107. "Catching Dangerous Rays," Newsweek, June 24, 1985, p. 69.

108. P. Robins, "The Sun and Skin Cancer," Bottom Line, March 30, 1984, pp. 11-12.

109. "Safety Belt Sense," Age Page, Washington, D.C. : U.S. Government Printing Office, 1983.

110. L. Gannon, "Who Needs A Seat Belt?" Reader's Digest, August, 1988, pp. 105-109.

111. "Auto Safety: More States Buckle Up." Time, January 20, 1986, p. 25.

112. J.A. Seamonds, "Seat-Belt Laws Aren't Deflating Those Air Bags," U.S. News and World Report, October 21, 1985, p. 55.

Notes to Chapter 4

113. K.R. Pelletier, Longevity: Fulfilling Our Biological Potential. New York: Dell, 1981, pp. 253-254.

114. R.S. Paffenbarger, "A Natural History of Athleticism and Cardiovascular Health," Journal of American Medical Association, Vol. 252, July, 1984, pp. 491-495.

115. Health People 2000, 1991, p. 55.

116. Indeed, some contend that the goal of a daily or weekly regimen of vigorous exercise is not necessary and, in fact, not achievable by most of us. For example, Bryant A. Stamford and Porter Shimer, in Fitness Without Exercise (New York: Warner Books, 1990) suggest that a more moderate and

relaxed approach involving ordinary tasks makes better sense and may have more lasting effects than exhaustive aerobic workouts.

117. William Rakowski and Vincent Mor, "The Association of Physical Activity With Mortality Among Older Adults in The Longitudinal Study of Aging (1984-1988)," Journal of Gerontology, Vol. 47, No. 4, pp. M122-129, 1992.

118. "Exercise Can Benefit Everyone," Perspective in Health Promotion and Aging, Vol. 6, No. 2, 1991, p.1.

119. Vic Sussman, "Muscle Bound," U.S. News & World Report, May 20, 1991, pp. 85-87.

120. Quoted in: Jane E. Brody, "The Trend Toward Inactivity Continues With The Unkindest Cut of All: Children's Fitness," The New York Times, February 8, 1993, p. B7.

121. Dr. Paul Z. Siegel, quoted in: Jane E. Brody, "The Trend Toward Inactivity Continues With the Unkindest Cut Of All: Children's Fitness," The New York Times, February 3, 1993, p. B7.

122. A. Toufexis, "The Shape of the Nation," Time, October 7, 1985, pp. 60-61.

123. H. Salisbury, A Journey For Our Times, New York: Harper & Row, 1984.

124. R. Paffenbarger, New England Journal of Medicine, March, 1986.

125. Ralph S. Paffenberger, et al, "The Association of Changes in Physical-Activity Level And Other Lifestyle Characteristics With Mortality Among Men," The New England Journal of Medicine, Vol. 328, February 25, 1993, pp. 538-545.

126. Those who have managed to get into shape and then abandon their program of regular exercise pay a heavy price. They soon discover that their fitness level quickly erodes, and before long they are once again out of shape. Studies show that even Olympic and college athletes who stop training when their competitive careers end, revert to having the same risk of heart disease as people who never exercised at all.

127. William Pollin and R.T. Ravenholt, "Tobacco Addiction and Tobacco Mortality," Journal of the American Medical Association, Vol. 252, November 23/30, 1984, pp. 2849-2854

128. Growing pubic concern over the hazards of smoking is now being reflected in divorce battles involving children. The early 1990s saw several cases of estranged parents invoking secondhand smoke as a point of contention in custody cases, nearly all involving children with respiratory ailments such as asthma and allergies. The typical outcome in such cases has been a court order prohibiting smoking around the child, violation of which could result in a jail sentence or other punishment. Indications are that smoking may become a significant factor in custodial disputes.

129. Lowell Ponte, "Deadly Mixers: Alcohol and Tobacco," Reader's Digest, April, 1985, pp. 53-56.

130. It is not always easy to institute such prohibitions. Sullivan (see Reference section) described the efforts of a school board member in a high-producing tobacco county in North Carolina who proposed that teachers and students be prohibited from smoking in school buildings. The proposal was approved by the board, but their decision lasted only one month. Resentful tobacco farmers threatened to retaliate by killing a $30 million school bond issue. The board then retreated, allowing school employees to smoke.

131. The Center for Disease Control estimated that about 750,000 cancer deaths were avoided or postponed over the last two decades because of people quitting or not starting to smoke in the first place. The Surgeon General's office estimates that 85 percent of lung cancer mortality could have been avoided if individuals had never taken up smoking. Unlike other types of cancer, lung cancer often fails to respond to treatment.

132. Lynn Langway, et al., "Showdown On Smoking," Newsweek, June 16, 1983, pp. 60-67.

133. Cindy L. Jajich, Adrian M. Ostfel, and Daniel H. Freeman, "Smoking and Coronary Heart Disease Mortality in the Elderly," Journal of the American Medical Association, Vol. 232, November 23/30, 1984, pp. 2831-2834.

134. Jean Seligman, et al., "Women Smokers: The Risk Factor," Newsweek, November 25, 1985, pp. 76-78.

135. Graham A. Colditz, et al., <u>New England Journal of Medicine</u>, April 14, 1988, pp. 937-41.

136. Karen F. Allen, et al, "Teenage Tobacco Use: Data Estimates From the Teenage Attitudes and Practices Survey, United States, 1989," Advance data from vital and health statistics, No. 224, February 1, 1993, Hyatsville, MD: National Center for Health Statistics, 1992.

137. <u>Journal of the American Medical Association</u>, December 11, 1991.

138. "Snuff Use Increases Despite Dangers," <u>Health Scene</u>, Hospital Corporation of America, North Florida Regional Medical Center, Gainesville, Florida, Fall, 1992, p. 2.

139. <u>New England Journal of Medicine</u>, January 30, 1992.

140. Joanne Lipman, "Media Content Is Linked to Cigarette Ads," <u>The Wall Street Journal</u>, January 30, 1992, p. B5.

141. Eben Shapiro, "Trend Toward Quitting Smoking Slows As Discount Cigarettes Gain Popularity," <u>The Wall Street Journal</u>, April 1, 1993.

142. Christopher Sullivan, "Health Advocates Challenge Tradition," <u>Gainesville Sun</u>, February 2, 1992, pp. 1G & 6G.

143. Hal Kane, "Putting Out Cigarettes," <u>World Watch</u>, September\October, 1992, p. 34.

144. L. Ponte, "Deadly Mixers: Alcohol and Tobacco," 1985, p. 53.

145. <u>Healthy People 2000</u>, 1991, p. 164.

146. Arthur Schatzkin, et. al, <u>New England Journal of Medicine</u>, May 1987.

147. Walter C. Willet, <u>New England Journal of Medicine</u>, May, 1987.

148. Ann Misch, "Richer Diets Risk Breast Cancer," <u>World Watch</u>, November/December, 1992, p. 36.

149. As Misch (1992) notes, Third World women are at even greater risk. In many of their countries the necessary diagnostic and treatment technologies are not available. Even if they were, most of the women could not afford

them. Hence, prevention, especially through dietary changes, may be the easiest and most common sense approach to the problem (p. 36).

150. Michael Waldholz, "Many Women With Breast Cancer Fail To Get Best Possible Care, Studies Find," The Wall Street Journal, December 26, 1991, p. B3. Studies reported in that week's Journal of the American Medical Association.

151. Trisha Thompson, "Wine, Women...and Questions, Redbook. June, 1992, pp. 74-77.

152. This lends some support to the theory that alcohol protects the heart by raising levels of beneficial high-density lipoprotein (HDL) cholesterol, which helps flush coronary arteries of fatty deposits. French researcher Martine Seifneur and her colleagues reported in 1990 that drinking one to three glasses of red wine each day significantly lowers artery-clogging, low-density lipoprotein (LDL) cholesterol, while elevating "good" high-density lipoprotein cholesterol (HDL). Red wine contains a chemical—**resveratrol**—derived from the wine grape skins, that appears to help lower LDL and raise good HDL.

153. Associated Press, "Drinkers Pay Warnings Little Heed, Studies Say," Gainesville Sun, November 11, 1991.

154. A methodological problem here involves the difficulty of untangling and assigning different weights to the various reasons people give for changing their drinking and driving habits.

Notes to Chapter 5

155. R.S. Lazaurus and J.B. Cohne, "Environmental Stress," in I. Altman and J.F. Wohlwill (Editors), Human Behavior and Environment, New York: Plenum, Vol. 22, 1977, pp. 89-127.

156. Mae Rudolph, "City Stress: Learning to Live in Condition Red," New York Magazine, Vol. 5, December 18/25, 1972, pp. 50-54.

157. T. Wilding, "Is Stress Making You Sick?" America's Health, Vol. 6, 1984, pp. 2-5.

158. Ibid.

159. Subsequently he and a colleague further refined this instrument which then became the widely used Holmes-Rahe scale.

160. Kenneth Lamott, "What To Do When Stress Signs Say You're Killing Yourself," Today's Health, Vol. 53, January, 1975, pp. 30-32, 59-60.

161. Henry Dreher, "Do You Have A Type-C (Cancer-Prone) Personality?" Redbook, May, 1988, pp. 108-109, 158-159.

162. Joan Arehart-Treichel, "Can Your Personality Kill You?" New York, November 28, 1977, pp. 62-67.

163. S.C. Kobasa, "Stressful Life Events, Personality, and Health: A Prospective Study," Journal of Personality and Social Psychology, Vol. 37, 1979, pp. 1-11.

164. S.C. Kobasa, "Hardiness and Health: A Prospective Study," Journal of Personality and Social Psychology, Vol. 42, 1982, pp. 168-177.

165. S.C. Kobasa, R.R. J. Hilker, and S.R. Maddi, "Who Stays Healthy Under Stress?" Journal of Occupational Medicine, Vol. 21, 1979, pp. 595-598.

166. D.T. Lykken, "Fearlessness: Its Carefree Charm and Deadly Risks," Psychology Today, Vol. 16, 1982, pp. 20-28.

167. In a later chapter we shall note that one characteristic of centenarians, people who live to be 100 years of age or older, is this sense of commitment, or involvement.

168. H. Selye, Stress Without Distress, New York: Signet, 1974, p. 66.

169. John F. Brantner, "Death and the Self," in Betty R. Green and Donald P. Irish (Editors), Death Education: Preparation for Living, Cambridge, MA: Schenkman Publishing Col, 1981, p. 23.

170. One American hostage in Iran was reported to have achieved some sense of control over his environment by purposely saving a small portion of each of his meals. Then, when anyone came into his cell, he would offer them some food. In a way, he gave himself the role of a host who had the power and the privilege to welcome visitors to his "abode."

171. Neal Krause, "Stress and Coping: Reconceptualizing the Role of Locus of Control Beliefs," Journal of Gerontology, Vol. 41, September, 1986, pp. 617-622. Interestingly, this study found that elderly persons with **extreme** internal and external locus of control beliefs were more vunerable to the deleterious effects of life stress than those with **moderate** control beliefs.

172. M. Pines, "Psychological Hardiness: The Role of Challenge in Health," Psychology Today, Vol. 14, 1980, pp. 34-44.

173. B.R. Strickland, "Internal-External Expectancies and Health-Related Behaviors," Journal of Consulting and Clinical Psychology, Vol. 46, 1978, pp. 1192-1211.

174. M.E.P. Seligman, Helplessness, San Francisco, CA: Freeman, 1975.

175. S.H. Croog and S,. Levine, The Heart Patient Recovers, New York: Human Science, 1971.

176. M. Seeman and T.E. Seeman, "Health Behavior and Personal Autonomy: A Longitudinal Study of the Sense of Control in Illness," Journal of Health and Social Behavior, Vol. 24, 1983, pp. 144-160.

177. G. Engel, "Emotional Stress and Sudden Death," Psychology Today, Vol. 11, 1977, pp. 153-154.

178. David Monagan, "Fatal Emotions," Reader's Digest, May, 1986 (condensed from Discover, January, 1986, New York: Time, Inc.), pp. 123-126.

Notes to Chapter 6

179. Quoted in: "Stress in Perspective," The Royal Bank Newsletter, Vol. 70, January/February, 1989, pp. 1-4.

180. M. Pines, "Psychological Hardiness: the Role of Challenge to Health," Psychology Today, Vol. 14, 1980, pp. 34-44.

181. Ibid.

182. Ibid. p. 40.

183. Nan Lin and Walter M. Ensel, "Life Stress and Health: Stressors and Resources," <u>American Sociological Review</u>, Vol. 54, June, 1989, pp. 382-399.

184. W.B. Cannon, "Voodoo Death," <u>American Anthropologist</u>, Vol. 44, 1942, pp. 169-181.

185. M. Pines, 1980.

186. D.C. McClelland, in G. Serban (Editors), <u>Sources of Stress in the Drive for Power</u>, New York: Plenum, 1976.

187. In McClelland's view, the behavior of persons who are high on the need for power but whose expressed motivation is inhibited, and therefore they are under power stress, closely resemble the Type A personality on a variety of characteristics—aggressive, competitive, argumentative, etc.

188. M. Pines, 1980.

189. C. Wallis, "Stress: Can We Cope?" <u>Time</u>, Vol. 121, June 6, 1983, pp. 48-54.

190. "Jobs Where Stress Is Most Severe," <u>U.S. News & World Report</u>. September 5, 1983, pp. 45-46.

191. Blair Wheaton, "Life Transitions, Role Histories, and Mental Health," <u>American Sociological Review</u>, Vol. 55, April, 1990, pp. 209-223.

192. She defines chronic stress as "continuous and persistent conditions in the social environment resulting in a problematic level of demand on the individual's capacity to perform adequately in social roles." (p. 210).

193. B.S. Dohrenwend, et al., "Exemplification of a Method For Scaling Life Events: The PERI Life Events Scale," <u>Journal of Health and Social Behavior</u>, Vol. 19, 1978, pp. 205-229.

194. J. Isherwood, "The Study of Life Event Stress," <u>New Zealand Psychologist</u>, Vol. 10, 1981, pp. 71-79.

195. "Stress Without Distress: How to Cope," 1984, <u>America's Health</u>, pp. 6-7.

196. "Making the Most of Time," <u>The Royal Bank Newsletter</u>, Vol. 67 January/February, 1986, pp. 1-4.

197. Ardis Whitman, "Secret Joys of Solitude," <u>Reader's Digest</u>, 1984.

198. "Spending Your Time," <u>The Royal Bank Newsletter</u>, Vol. 67, July/August, 1984, pp. 1-4. See also: "The Place of Recreation," Vol. 73, January/February, 1992, pp. 1-4.

199. Claudia Wallis, "Stress: Can We Cope?" <u>Time</u>, June 6, 1983, pp. 48-54.

200. Carol Tavris, <u>Anger: The Misunderstood Emotion</u>, New York: Simon and Schuster, 1982.

201. Redford B. Williams, quoted in: Marion Long, "Anger: How Mad Is Bad?" <u>Family Weekly</u>, January 25, 1983, pp. 4-5, 7.

202. Raymond B. Flannery, Jr. <u>Becoming Stress-Resistant</u>. New York: Continuum, 1991.

Notes to Chapter 7

203. L.F. Berkman, and S.L Syme, "Social Networks, Host Resistance, and Mortality: A Nine-Year Follow-Up Study of Almeda County Residents." <u>American Journal of Epidemiology</u>, Vol. 109, 1979, pp. 186-204.

204. W. D. Rees, and S. G. Lutkins, "Mortality of Bereavement," <u>British Medical Journal</u>, Vol. 4, 1967, pp. 13-16.

205. J. J. Lynch, <u>The Broken Heart: The Medical Consequences of Loneliness</u>. New York: Basic Books, 1977, p. 56.

206. E. Durkheim, E., <u>Suicide</u>. Translated by J. A. Spaulding, and G. Simpson, Glencoe, IL: Free Press, 1951.

207. G. Engel, "Emotional Stress and Sudden Death." <u>Psychology Today</u>, Vol. 11, 1977, pp. 114, 118, 153.

208. "Broken Heart Syndrome." <u>Newsweek</u>, October 23, 1967, p. 92.

209. G. Dullea, "Begin's Decline Not Surprising to Professionals," <u>Gainesville Sun</u>, September 14, 1983, p. 1B.

210. Menachem Begin died of heart trouble in 1992 at the age of 78, after more than eight years of near hermitic retirement.

211. C. M. Parkes, <u>Bereavement: Studies of Grief in Adult Life</u>, New York: International Universities Press, 1972, p.17.

212. S. J., Schleifer, et al., "Suppression of Lymphocyte Stimulation Following Bereavement." <u>Journal of the American Medical Association</u>, Vol. 250 (July, 1983), pp. 374-377.

213. B.S. Bender, et al., "Absolute Peripheral Blood Lymphocyte Count and Subsequent Mortality of Elderly Men," JAGS, Vol. 1986, pp. 649-654.

214. J.R. Brown and G.A. Stoudemire, "Normal and Pathological Grief," <u>Journal of the American Medical Association</u>, Vol. 250, July 1983, pp. 378-382.

215. Knowledge about the functioning of the immune system and how it is affected by the altered biochemistry of the body due to the stress of grief is slowly growing. We do know that bereaved individuals become extremely susceptible to bacterial, fungal and viral infections, and that the immune mechanism fails to detect cells altered via exposure to oncogenic viruses or environmental carcinogens.

216. M. Young, B. Benjamin, and C. Wallis, "The Mortality of Widowers," <u>The Lancet</u>, August, 1963, pp. 454-456.

217. B. Kutner, et al., <u>Five-Hundred Over Sixty</u>, New York: Russell Sage Foundation, 1956, p. 63.

218. P. Townsen, <u>The Family Life of Old People</u>, London: Routledge and Kegan, 1957.

219. K. J. Helsig, M. Szklo, G. W. Comstock, "Factors Associated with Mortality After Widowhood," <u>American Journal of Public Health</u>, Vol. 17, 1981, pp. 803-809.

220. Despite the differences in death rates, it was found that widowed men and married men generally died of the same causes, such as heart disease, cancer, and other ailments.

221. J. Greenberg, "Marriage and Mortality," <u>New York Times</u>, August, 1981, pp. 1A, 16A.

222. K. Helsig, et al., 1981, p. 809.

223. Z. S. Blau, <u>Aging in a Changing Society</u>, 2nd ed., New York: Franklin Watts, 1981.

224. F.M. Berardo, "Widowhood Status in the Unites States: Perspectives on a Neglected Aspect of the Family Life Cycle," <u>The Family Coordinator</u>, Vol. 17, 1968, pp. 191-203. See also: "Survivorship and Social Isolation: The Case of the Aged Widower," Vol. 19, 1970, pp. 11-25.

225. K.J. Helsing, et al., 1981, p. 808.

226. House (1983) cites research which suggests that social support can operate across species. Included is evidence that pets can enhance the well-being of people and, conversely, people can be effective sources of social support for animals as well.

227. To achieve this end, certain conceptual and methodological problems associated with research on informal support networks need to be addressed. See: Russell A. Ward, "Informal Networks and Well-Being in Later Life: A Research Agenda," <u>The Gerontologist</u>, Vol. 25, 1985, pp. 51-61.

228. James Harrison, "Warning: The Male Sex Role May Be Dangerous to Your Health," <u>Journal of Social Issues</u>, Vol. 34, Winter, 1978, pp. 65-86.

229. Edward Dolnick, "Why Women Live Longer Than Men," printed in <u>Reader's Digest</u>, 1991, pp. 157-160, as a condensed version of an original article in <u>Health</u>, July/August, 1991, published by Hippocrates Partners, Sausalito, California. The original author may be Deborah Wingard.

230. Kate Zernike, "The Bell Tolls For the Future Merry Widow," The New York Times, 2006.

231. Three major factors contribute to the growing excess of widows in the United States: (a) mortality among females is lower than among males; therefore larger numbers of women survive to advanced years; (b) wives are typically younger than their husbands and, consequently, have a greater

probability of outliving them; and (c) among the widowed, remarriage rates are considerable lower for women than for men.

232. J. Fox, L. Bulusa, and L. Kinlen, "Mortality and Age Differences in Marriage." Journal of Gerontology, Vol. 39, 1979, pp. 117-120.

233. D. Foster, L. Klinger-Vartabedian, and L. Wispe, "Male Longevity and Age Differences Between Spouses." Journal of Gerontology, Vol. 39, 1979, pp, 117-120.

234. W. McKain, "Retirement Marriage," Storrs Agricultural Experiment Station Monograph 3, Storrs: University of Connecticut, 1969.

235. J.J. Lynch, "Doctor's Warning: Being Single Can Be Hazardous to Your Health." Harper's Bazaar, October, 1978, pp. 182-183.

236. However, a survey by the Michigan Cancer Foundation of over 59,000 cancer cases suggests that marital status has no effect on the chances of contracting cancer, but that once the disease occurs, marriage is a protective factor **for survivorship**. The study also found that the relationship between cancer and marital status differs dramatically depending on sex, race, and type of cancer. For example, single black males had by far the highest incidence of lung, colon and pancreas cancer of all the groups studied. (Mark Fritz, "Study: Singles Are a Higher Cancer Risk," Gainesville Sun, November 5, 1985, p. 8D.)

237. R.B. Case, A. J. Moss, N. Case, M. McDermott, S. Eberly, "Living alone after myocardial Infraction. Impact on prognosis," Journal of the American Medical Association, Vol. 267, No. 4, January, 1992, pp. 515-519.

238. J.J. Lynch, The Broken Heart: The Medical Consequences of Loneliness. New York: Basic Books, 1977.

239. Robert H. Coombs, "Marital Status and Personal Well-Being: A Literature Review," Family Relations, Vol. 40, January, 1991, pp. 97-102.

240. Duane F. Alwin and Philip E. Converse, "Living Arrangements, Social Integration, and Psychological Well-Being," Paper presented at the annual meetings of the Midwest Sociological Association, Chicago, April, 1984.

241. Duane F. Alwin, Philip E. Converse, and Steven S. Martin, "Living Arrangements and Social Integration," <u>Journal of Marriage and the Family</u>, Vol. No. 2, 1985, pp. 319-334.

242. This is especially the case for men, who appear to benefit the most from marriage. For example, in a study conducted at the University of California at San Francisco the lifestyles of over 7600 adults were analyzed to determine whether living arrangments were linked to their eventual length of survival. The analysis showed men between the ages of 45 and 64 who lived alone, or with someone other than a spouse, were twice as like to die within 10 years as men of the same age who resided with their wives. For women there was no direct correlation between marriage and longevity—however, a social support system was associated with greater longevity.

243. Leo Buscaglia, <u>Loving Each Other: The Challenge of Human Relationships</u>, Thorofare, NJ: SLACK Incorporated, 1984. Distributed by Holt, Rinehart and Winston.

Notes to Chapter 8

244. R. Hodgson and P. Miller, <u>Self-Watching. Addiction. Habits, Compulsions: What To Do About Them</u>, New York: Facts on File, 1982.

245. S. Cohen, "Fitness as in Wellness," <u>Newsweek</u>, 1987.

246. Ray Hodgson and Peter Miller, <u>Selfwatching: Addictions, Habits, Compulsions: What To Do About Them</u>, New York: Facts on File, 1982.

247. W. Goodman and L. Prout, "Good News About Bad Habits," <u>Newsweek</u>, September 13, 1982, p. 86.

248. M. Seeman and T.E. Seeman, "Health Behavior and Personal Autonomy: A Longitudinal Study of the Sense of Control in Illness," <u>Journal of Health and Social Behavior</u>, Vol. 24, 1983, pp. 144-160.

249. M. Pines, "Psychological Hardiness: The Role of Challenge in Health," <u>Psychology Today</u>, Vol. 14, 1980, pp. 34-44.

250. Hodgson and Miller, 1982, p. 11.

251. G.A. Marlatt and J.R. Gordon (Editors), <u>Relapse Prevention</u>, New York: Guilford Press, 1985.

252. Stanton Peele, "Out of the Habit Trap," <u>American Health: Fitness of Body and Mind</u>, September\October, 1983, pp. 180-184.

253. C. Leerdhsen, et al., "Unite and Conquer," <u>Newsweek</u>, February 5, 1990, pp. 50-55.

254. S. Schacter, in Goodman and Prout, p. 86.

255. Edwin Kiester, Jr., and Sally Valente Kiester, "A Clean Break With Bad Habits," <u>Reader's Digest</u>, November, 1989, pp. 165-170.

256. L.W. Green, "Evaluation and Measurement: Some Dilemmas for Health Education," <u>American Journal of Public Health</u>, Vol. 67, February, 1977, p. 158.

257. J. Bruhn, "Creating Risk Sensitive Persons: The Roles of Choice and Chance in Staying Healthy," <u>Southern Medical Journal</u>, Vol. 81 (1988), pp. 624-629.

258. M. Rokeach, <u>Understanding Human Values: Individual and Societal</u>, New York: The Free Press, 1979.

259. K.A. Wallston and B.S. Wallston, "Health Locus of Control Scales," in H.M. Lefcourt (Editor), <u>Research With the Locus of Control Construct</u>, New York: Academic Press, 1983, pp. 189-243.

260. Peele, 1983, p. 181.

261. Ibid, p. 183.

Notes to Chapter 9

262. U. S. Department of Health and Human Services, <u>Geographic Patterns in the Risk of Dying and Associated Factors, Ages 35-74 Years</u>, Hyattsville, MD: National Center for Health Statistics, 1980, pp. 47-57.

263. Victor R. Fuchs, "A Tale of Two Cities," in Peter Conrad and Rocelle Kern (Editors), The Sociology of Health and Illness, 3rd Edition, New York: St. Martin's Press, 1992, pp. 57-59.

264. C.Goldscheider, "The Social Inequality of Death." In E. Shneidman (Ed.), Death: Current Perspectives, 3rd ed., Palo Alto, CA: Mayfield, 1984, p. 38.

265. Sandra Blakeslee, "Studies Uncover Disparity Among Kidney Recipients," The Gainesville Sun, January 24, 1989, p. 2A.

266. Bernard Friedman, Ronald J. Ozminkowski, and Zachary Taylor, "Excess Demand and Patient Selection for Heart and Liver Transplantation." Health Economics Worldwide, 1991, pp. 161-186.

267. Charlotte A. Schoenborn, Jackline L. Vickerie, and Eve Powell-Griner, "Health Charactistics of Adults 55 Years of Age and Over: United States, 2000-2003." Advance data from Vital and Health Statistics: No 370. Yattsville, MD: National Center for Health Statistics, 2006.

268. Susan P. Baker, "Injuries in America: A National Disaster," in Russell C. Maulitz (Editor), Unnatural Causes: The Three Leading Killer Diseases in America, New Brunswick, New Jersey: Rutgers University Press, 1989, pp. 135-145.

269. Schwirian, K. P., and LaGreca, A. J. 1971, December, "An Ecological Analysis of Urban Mortality Rates." Social Science Quarterly, pp. 574-587.

270. A. Toufexis, "Cardiology City, U.S.S.R." Time, November 28, 1983, p. 70.

271. C. Wallis, "Stress: Can We Cope?" Time, June 6, 1983, pp. 48-54.

272. M. Rudolph, "City Stress: Learning to Live in Condition Red," New Yorker, Vol. 5, 1972, pp. 50-54.

273. C. Perrow, Normal Accidents: Living with High-Risk Technologies. New York: Basic Books, 1984.

274. Lee Clarke, Acceptable Risk? Making Decisions in a Toxic Environment, Berkeley: University of California Press, 1989.

275. <u>Healthy People 2000</u>, 1991, p. 392.

276. Amasa B. Ford, "Casualties of Our Time," <u>Science</u>, Vol. 167, January 16, 1970, pp. 256-263.

Notes to Chapter 10

277. Gina Kolata, "Questions Raised on FDA's Authority to Protect Public," <u>Gainesville Sun</u>, January 26, 1992.

278. "Give The FDA Watchdogs Some Tough New Teeth," <u>USA Today</u>, February 4, 1992, p. 8A.

279. Gardiner Harris, "Congressional Investigators Are Critical of F.D.A.'s Efforts to Detect Drug Dangers." The New Times, April 24th 2006, p. A12.

280. A.B. Ford, "Casualties Of Our Time," <u>Science</u>, Vol. 167, 1970, p. 260.

281. A. Toufexis, "Linking Drugs to the Dinner Table," <u>Time</u>, September 24, 1984, p. 77.

282. Ibid, p. 77.

283. The American public is little aware that diseased and contaminated cattle are regularly approved for consumption. See: Jeremy Rifkin, <u>Beyond Beef</u>, New York: Dutton, 1992. Much of this book deals with the environmental damage brought on by the spread of cattle ranching. Rifkin argues that a third of all the grain produced worldwide is fed to livestock, and that much of that grain should be used to feed hungry people.

284. F. Golden, "Heat Over Wood Burning." <u>Time</u>, Vol. 123, January 16, 1984, p. 67.

285. A. Trafford, "America's Diet Wars," <u>U.S. News & World Report</u>, January 20, 1986, pp. 62-66h.

286. Quoted in A. Trafford, "America's Diet Wars," 1986.

287. A high profile example was provided by the television talk show host Opra Winfrey. After following one of the more expensive liquid diet programs

she lost 67 pounds. To dramatize the loss, and her new, slim figure, she opened one of her shows by pulling a wagon containing 67 pounds of meat onto the set. She clearly was proud of her accomplishment, said she felt much better physically and psychologically than she had in years, and encouraged others to get their bodies back into shape. Unfortunately, the euphoria did not last very long. With months, Oprah has regained all of her lost weight, and much more. There was no way she could hide this sad reversal of circumstances, since she had to appear every weekday on national television to do her show.

288. Claude Bouchard, "Is Weight Fluctuation a Risk Factor?" The New England Journal of Medicine, Vol. 324, June 27, 1991, pp. 1887-1887.

289. Bouchard (1991) notes that the evidence that weight fluctuations in humans have health implications is meager and draws support primarily from animal studies. Hence, some scientists are skeptical of this *weight-cycling hypothesis* as it relates to human populations. Until better animal and epidemiologic studies are carried out, he cautions, one should be tentative in drawing specific conclusions.

290. L. Lissner, et al., "Variability of body weight and health outcomes in the Framingham population," The New England Journal of Medicine, Vol. 324, No. 26, June 27, 1991, pp. 1839-1844.

291. M. H. Brenner, "Estimating the Effects of Economic Change on National health and Social Well-Being," No. SPRT 98-198. Washington, D.C.: U. S. Government Printing Office, 1984.

292. "And the Poor Get Sicker." 1984, September, Scientific America, 251, p. 82.

293. C. Goldscheider, C., "The Social Inequality of Death," in E. Shneidman (Editor), Death: Current Perspectives, 3rd Edition, Palo Alto, CA: Mayfield, 1984, pp. 35-36.

294. W. Rinehart, A. Kols, and S.H. Moore, "Healthier Mothers and Children Through Family Planning," Population Reports, Series J, Vol. 12, No. 27, 1984.

295. Louis W. Sullivan, "Forward," <u>Healthy People 2000: National Health Promotion and Disease Prevention Objectives</u>, Washington, D.C.: U.S. Government Printing Office, 1991, p. v.

296. Nicholas Eberstadt, "America's Infant Mortality Problem: Parents," <u>The Wall Street Journal</u>, January 20, 1992.

297. Michael Waldholz, "Uninsured Infants Taken to Hospitals Get Fewer Services," <u>The Wall Street Journal</u>, December 18, 1991, p. B3. (see Paula Braverman and Jonathan Showstack, <u>Journal of the American Medical Association</u>.)

298. "Uninsured Patients More Likely to Die," <u>New York Times</u>, January 16, 1991. (team headed by Center's co-director, Jack Hadley)

299. Gary J. Young and Bruce B. Cohen, "Inequities in Hospital Care, the Massachusetts Experience," <u>Inquiry</u>, Vol. 23, No. 3, Fall, 1991, pp. 255-262.

300. Hilary Stout, "More Than 100 Hospitals Had High Death Rates in 1990," <u>Wall Street Journal</u>, June 11, 1992, p. B8.

Notes to Chapter 11

301. Herman E. Koenig, William E. Cooper, and James M. Falvey, "Engineering for Ecological, Sociological, and Economic Compatibility," <u>IEEE Transactions on Systems, Man, and Cybernetics</u>, Vol. SMC-2, No. 3, July, 1972, pp. 319-331.

302. William K. Stevens, "Rio: A Start on Managing What's Left of This Place," <u>New York Times</u>, May 31, 1992, p.6.

303. Two recent examples of such polemical attacks can be found in Ronald Bailey, <u>Eco-Scam: The False Prophets of Ecological Apocalypse</u>, New York: St. Martin's Press, 1993; Michael Fumento, <u>Science Under Siege: Balancing Technology and the Environment</u>, New York: Morrow, 1993.

304. Amasa B. Ford, "Casualties of Our Times," <u>Science</u>, Vol. 167, January 16, 1970, pp. 256-263.

305. John Carey, with Mary Hager, Patricia King, and Seth Zuckerman, "Beware 'Sick-Building' Syndrome," <u>Newsweek</u>, January 7, 1985, p. 58.

306. According to the U.S. Environmental Protection Agency (EPA), any substance that is explosive, corrosive, highly flammable or poisonous (or if it can become so by interacting with another substance), is hazardous. Among the common household products that fit this description are paint thinner, turpentine, varnish, insecticide, polish, charcoal lighter, auto fluids, glue, enamel, batteries, rust removal products and any other products. Hazardous products that are improperly disposed can create fires and explosions, can cause birth defects and other medical problems, and can be directly poisonous to humans and wildlife.

307. Establishing causality is always a scientific challenge. For example, it is generally agreed that **radon gas**, a product of radioactive decay of the uranium in rocks and soil, is a health hazard. Because it is invisible and odorless, it can accumulate silently in the home as it seeps through walls and openings. Exposure over time can eventually cause lung cancer. It is estimated that radon gas is responsible for between 5,000 and 20,000 deaths each year. However, it is especially carcinogenic when combined with smoking. Trying to establish their separate contributions to lung cancer then becomes much more problematic. (See: Terence Monmaney, with Mary Hager and Tony Emerson, "The Risk of Radon," <u>Newsweek</u>, September 26, 1988, p.69.

308. John S. Demott, "An Unending Search for Safety," <u>Time</u>, December 17, 1984, p. 35.

309. Michael R. Edelstein, <u>Contaminated Communities: The Social and Psychological Impacts of Residential Toxic Exposure</u>, Boulder, Colorado: Westview Press, 1988.

310. Ibid, p. 34.

311. Apparently there is a growing tendency for the large, multinational chemical companies to locate their more hazardous plants in developing nations to escape the more stringent safety regulations of their own countries.

312. Natalie Angler, "Hazards Of a Toxic Wasteland," <u>Time</u>, December 17, 1984, p. 33.

313. Robert Suro, "Abandoned Oil and Gas Wells Are Now Portals for Pollution," <u>New York Times</u>, May 3, 1992, p. 11.

314. Natalie Angler, 1984, p. 34.

315. Natalie Angler, 1984, p. 34.

316. Michael Brown, <u>Laying Waste</u>: <u>The Poisoning of America by Toxic Chem-icals,</u> New York: Pantheon Books, 1980.

317. Rachel Carson, <u>Silent Spring</u>, Boston: Houghton Mifflin, 1962.

318. Sharon Begley, with Gerald C. Lubenow, "Silent Spring Revisited," <u>News-week</u>, July 14, 1986, pp. 72-73.

319. It is a common argument among manufacturers that banning certain of their products is not worth the economic cost. For example, the EPA esti-mates that banning asbestos would save roughly 2000 lives over the next 15 years. Producers in turn estimate that the cost of replacing asbestos will be $2 billion dollars. They argue this is too high a price to pay to justify the ban. (See:Bill Powell, "The Case for Asbestos," <u>Newsweek</u>, September 29, 1986, pp. 40-41).

320. Mary S. Wolff, "Blood Levels of Organochlorine Residues and Risk of Breast Cancer," <u>Journal of the National Cancer Institute</u>, April 21, 1993, pp. Cited in Elyse Tanouye, "Breast Cancer, DDT Exposure Linked in Study," <u>The Wall Street Journal</u>, April 21, 1993, p. B5.

321. Begley, 1986, p. 73.

322. Frank Edward Allen, "One Man's Suffering Spurs Doctors to Probe Pesti-cide-Drug Link," <u>The Wall Street Journal</u>, October 14, 1991, p. A1, A4.

323. Allen, 1991, p. 4A.

324. "Too Much Fuss About Pesticides?" <u>Consumer Reports</u>, October, 1989, pp. 655-658.

325. Edelstein, 1988, pp. 191-92.

Notes to Chapter 12

326. "Wasted Health Care Dollars," <u>Consumer Reports</u> Vol. 57, July, 1992, pp. 435-448.

327. *Consumer Reports* traces the spiraling costs of medical care, fueled primarily by rapidly rising hospital and physician charges, to the advent in 1965 of the government-financed Medicare and Medicaid programs, which were designed to provide health insurance for the elderly.

328. For example, researchers have found high rates of unnecessary usage for back surgery, magnetic resonance imaging, prostate surgery, the more costly clot-busting drugs for heart attack victims, carpel tunnel syndrome (wrist ailment), tonsillectomy, and upper gastrointestinal x-rays.

329. Lani Luciano, "A Cure Your M.D. Won't Like," Money Magazine Extra, 1990, pp. 54-59.

330. Consumer Reports, July, 1992, pp. 445-447.

331. Julian Whitaker, "Treatments That Are More Lethal Than the Diseases They Treat," Wellness Today, A Special Supplement to Health and Healing, Potomac, MD: Phillips Publishing, July, 1992.

332. Robin Marantz Henig, "The Unkindest Cut of All: Unnecessary Operations Raise Costs, Risks to Patients," AARP Bulletin, Vol. 33, September, 1992, pp. 2 & 16.

333. Luciano, 1990, p. 56.

334. Ibid, p. 58.

335. "Pushing Drugs to Doctors," Consumer Reports, February, 1992, pp. 87-94.

336. Daniel Carlat, "Generic Smear Campaign," The New York Times, May 2006, p. A27.

337. Ethical guidelines adopted by the American Medical Association and the Pharmaceutical Manufacturers Association prohibited drug companies from offering gifts and physicians from accepting them. One strategy used by prescription-drug manufacturers side-step the intent of these guidelines was to shift promotional efforts to *patient* giveaways. (See, for example, Doug Podolsky and Richard J. Newman, "Prescription Prizes," *U.S. News & World Report*, March 29, 1993, pp. 56-60.

338. L.W. Green, "Determining the Impact and Effectiveness of Health Education As It Relates to Federal Policy," Health Education Monographs, Vol. 6, Supplement No. 1, 1978, pp. 28-66.

339. Ibid, p. 54.

340. Paul Krugman, "Death By Insurance," The New York Times, 2006

341. Godfrey M. Hochbaum, "Ethical Dilemmas in Health Education," Health Education, March-April, 1980, pp. 4-6.

342. Spyros Doxiadis, Ethical Dilemmas in Health Promotion, New York: Johy Wiley Sons, 1987, Reprinted 1990.

343. Jean Seligmann and Donna Foote, "Whose Baby Is It, Anyway?" Newsweek, October 28, 1991.

344. Sharon Begley *with* Elizabeth Roberts, "Dishing Up Gamma Rays," Newsweek, January 27, 1992, pp. 52-53.

345. Matt Clark, et al., "Is Caffeine Bad for You?" Newsweek, July 19, 1982, pp. 62-64.

346. Jane E. Brody, "Don't Panic. Before Worrying About All The Medical Studies, Take A Close Look At the Evidence," New York Times, February 24, 1993, p. B7.

347. Ibid, p. B7.

348. Melinda Beck, with Farai Chideya and Brynn Craffey, "More and More People Are Living to See 100," Newsweek, May 4, 1992.

349. Helen Cooper, "Scientists Study How Some Centenarians Have Managed to Stay Hale and Hearty," Wall Street Journal, November 12, 1992, pp. B1 & B16.

350. James Kilpatrick, Portland Oregonian, December 23, 1983. Quoted in Howard M. Leichter, Free To Be Foolish: Politics and Health Promotion in The United States and Great Britain, Princeton, New Jersey: Princeton University Press, 1991, p. 3.

351. Dan Beauchamp, "Life-Style, Public Health and Paternalism," in Spyros Doxiadis (Editor), Ethical Dilemmas In Health Promotion, New York: John Wiley & Sons, 1990, p.69.

352. E.G. Knox, "Personal and Public Health Care: Conflict, Congruence or Accomodation," in Spyros Doxiadis (Editor), Ethical Dilemmas in Health Promotion, New York: John Wiley & Sons, 1990, pp. 59-68.

Notes to Chapter 13

353. Sharon Begley, et al., "A Long Summer of Smog," Newsweek, August 29, 1988, pp. 46-48.

354. U. S. Department of Health and Human Services, Public Health Service, Healthy People 2000: National Health Promotion and Disease Prevention Objectives, Washington DC: U.S. Government Printing Office, 1991.

355. Ibid, p. 496.

356. Marilyn Chase, "High HIV Level Is Found in Study of Poor Youth," Wall Street Journal, November 5, 1991. Article based on current issue of the Journal of the American Medical Association.

357. Fred J. Hellinger, "Forecasting the Medical Care Costs of the HIV Epidemic: 1991-1994," Inquiry, Vol. 28, Fall, 1991, pp. 213-225.

358. R. Widdus, et al., "The Management of Risk in Sexually Transmitted Diseases," Daedalus, Vol. 119, Fall, 1991, pp. 177-191.

359. Healthy People 2000, 1991, p. 273.

360. Not surprisingly, accident records also show that males are more likely than females to experience unintentional injuries, and are more likely to die from them. Black males generally have the highest death rate of all groups encountering accidents.

361. Healthy People 2000, 1991, p. 13.

362. Potential life lost is typically defined in terms of some average length of productive life. For example, if we arbitraily set 65 years of age as the average length of a productive life, then a death at age 60, lets say, would result

in loss of five years of productive life; a death at age 20 would mean 45 years of potential life lost.

363. Lois A. Fingerhut, "Firearm Mortality Among Children, Youth, and Young Adults 1—34 Years of Age, Trends and Current Status: United States, 1985-90," Advanced Data From Vital and Health Statistics; No. 231, Hyattsville, Maryland: National Center for Health Statistics, 1993.

364. The 1990's saw the emergence of another from of violence, car-hijacking, in which automobile drivers are suddenly confronted and threatened at the point of a gun to either give up their vehicles or be shot.

365. Healthy People 2000, 1991, pp. 236-237.

366. Erik Eckholm, "Gun Manufacturers Strive to Reverse Recent Slump in Sales," Gainesville Sun, March 15, 1992, p. 1G.

367. Don Terry, "A River of Illegal Guns Floods American Neighborhoods," Gainesville Sun, March 15, 1992, p. 1G.

368. Charles M. Callahan, "Urban High School Youth and Handguns," Journal of the American Medical Association, Vol. 267, June 10, 1992, pp. 3038-3042.

369. C. Everett Koop and George D. Lundberg, "Violence in America: A Public Health Emergency," Journal of the AMerican Medcial Association, Vol. 267, June 10, 1992, pp. 3075-3076.

370. Katherine Bishop, "New Gun Law Sets Off Debate in California," New York Times, January 2, 1992, p. A8.

371. Mark L. Rosenberg, "Violence Is a Public Health Problem," in Russell C. Maulitz (Editor), Unnatural Causes: The Three Leading Killer Diseases in America, New Brunswick, NJ: Rutgers University Press, 1989, p. 150.

372. Colin Loftin, et al., "Effects of Restrictive Licensing of Handguns on Homicide and Suicide in the District of Columbia," New England Journal of Medicine, Vol. 325, December, 1991, pp. 1615-1620. Also cited in Ron Winslow, "Study Links Drop in Firearm Deaths to Handgun Law," Wall Street Journal, December 5, 1991.

373. Peter M. Marzuk, et al., "The Effect of Access to Lethal Methods of Injury on Suicide Rates," Archives of General Psychiatry, Vol. 49, June, 1992, pp. 451-458.

374. Paul Cotton, "Gun-Associated Violence Increasingly Viewed as Public Health Challenge," Journal of the American Medical Association, Vol. 267, March, 1992, pp. 1171-1172.

375. Koop and Lundberg, 1992, p. 3076

376. Garen Wintemute, "Motor Vehicles or Firearms: Which Takes a Heavier Toll?" Journal of the American Medical Association, Vol. 269, No. 17, May 5, 1993, p. 2213.

Notes to Chapter 14

377. Cynthia P. Green, "The Environment and Population Growth: Decade for Action," Population Reports, Series M, No. 10. Baltimore, MD: Johns Hopkins University, Population Information Program, May 1992, p. 2.

378. Narendra P. Sharma, "Managing The World's Forests: Looking for Balance Between Conservation and Development," The Key Reporter, Phi Beta Kappa, Summer, 1992, pp. 7-12.

379. Sharma, "Managing the World's Forests", p. 7.

380. The Population Institute, Annual Report, Washington, D.C., 1991.

381. Cynthia P. Green, 1992, p. 4.

382. As noted earlier, not everyone shares these predictions for future environmental disasters. Several skeptics have argued that such conclusions are not warranted by the data at hand. Illustrative of this skeptical challenge are: Ronald Bailey, *Eco-Scam: The False Prophets of Ecological Apocalypse*, New York: St. Martin;s Press, 1993; and, Michael Fumento, *Science Under Siege: Balancing Technology and the Environment*, New York: Morrow, 1993. A sympathetic review of these books can be found in S. Fred Singer, "Environmental Fear-Mongers Exposed," *The Wall Street Journal*, April 28, 1993.

383. Hal Kane, "Fishing for Trouble," <u>World Watch</u>, November\December, 1992, pp. 33-35.

384. Joseph A. McFalls, Jr., "Population: A Lively Introduction," <u>Population Bulletin</u>, Vol. 46, No. 2, Washington, DC: Populaton Reference Bureau, October, 1991, p. 30.

385. Population Institute, <u>Annual Report</u>, 1991.

386. World Population Institute, <u>Annual Report</u>, 1992.

387. Cynthia P. Green, 1992, p. 4.

388. Ibid, p. 5.

389. A step in this direction was taken following the 1992 Earth Summit in Rio. Some months after those meetings in Rio de Janeiro, representatives of the industrialized and developing countries agreed on the composition and powers of a Sustainable Development Committee, charged with monitoring how well governments meet the promises made at the summit. However, the Committee lacks the power to force governments to honor their pledges. Instead it will rely on publicity and political pressure to make nations comply with commitments contained in Agenda 21, which is a blueprint for correcting current environmental problems, and assurances that future economic developments will be environmentally sound.

390. Lester R. Brown, Christopher Flavin, and Sandra Postel. <u>Saving The Planet</u>, How to Shape an Environmentally Sustainable Global Economy, New York: W.W. Norton, 1991.

391. Daniel Callahan, <u>The Tyranny of Survival, and Other Pathologies of Civilized Life</u>, New York: Macmillian, 1973.

392. Lester R. Brown, "Launching the Environmental Revolution," in Lester R. Brown, et al., <u>State of the World, 1992</u>, A Worldwatch Institute Report on Progress Towards a Sustainable Society, New York: W.W. Norton, 1992, pp. 175-190.

393. Lester R. Brown, "Launching the Environmental Revolution," 1992, p. 190.

Notes to Chapter 15

394. G. Will, 1984, "Social Disease in America." Gainesville Sun, May 1, 5A.

395. James J. Kilpatrick, "Almost Everything Can Kill Us," The Florida Times Union, April 24, 1984, p. A-ll.

396. Carl Rowan, "The Hard Route to Living Long," St. Petersburg Times, December 28, 1984, p. 2B.

397. Daniel O. Haney, "Getting Out of Bed May Be The Riskiest Act of the Day," Sunday Advocate, Baton Rouge, Louisiana, March 10, 1991, p. 7A.

398. Daniel Q. Haney, "Dream Hard On Your Heart, Study Suggests," The Gainesville Sun, February, 4, 1993, pp. 1A & 4A. Story derived from a report in The New England Journal of Medicine, February, 1993.

399. "Dangerous When Dead," Newsweek, August 27, 1990, p. 55.

400. Study conducted by Patricia Hebert, Harvard Medical School, and reported in Newsweek, November 25, 1991, p. 62.

401. Densie Webb, "Eating Well," The New York Times, October 21, 1992.

402. Ibid.

403. Ibid, citing nutritionist Dr. Susan Male Smith.

404. Lewis Grizzard, "Things That Go Bump In the 80's," Gainesville Sun, 1984, "What You Don't Know Won't Kill You," Gainesville Sun, 1985.

405. W.E. Wilbanks, "The New Obscenity." Vital Speeches of the Day. Address delivered as Belton High School, Texas, May, 1988.

406. A. Levine, "America's Addiction to Addictions," U.S. News & World Report, February 5, 1990, pp. 62-63.

407. Some have serious reservations about this expansion of the list of addictive behaviors and argue that it encourages people to attribute their shortcomings to victimization by others, thereby absolving themselves from all responsibility. See: Joseph Epstein, "Today's Professional Victims," New York Times Magazine, July 2, 1989.

408. Wilbanks, 1989, p. 103.

409. The reader may recall the extreme case of Howard Hughes, the recluse millionaire, who attempted to avoid all physical contact with others out of a pathological fear of becoming contaminated with other people's germs.

410. "Bad Apples. Alar: Not Gone, Not Forgotten," Consumer Reports, May, 1989, p. 291.

411. Elizabeth Whelan, "Nosophobia: How Fear of Disease Is Making Us Sick," in Bottom Line Year Book 1993, by the Editors of Bottom Line, New York: Boardroom Reports, Inc., 1992, pp. 19-20.

412. Again, the situation is often provoked by inconsistent or contradictory reports from all sides. For example, while some were claiming the threats to life posed by Alar, others were countering that such statements were alarmist and inaccurate. For example, during the scare over this pesticide reached worldwide proportions, a British government advisory committee, after reviewing the test data on Alar and UDMH, reached the unequivocal conclusion that: "Even for children consuming the maximum quantities of apples and apple juice, subjected to the maximum treatment with daminozide, there is no risk." Quoted in: Robert James Bidinotto, "The Great Apple Scare," Reader's Digest, December, 1990, p. 57.

413. Susan Baur, Hypochondria: Woeful Imaginings, University of California Press, 1988, has observed how we increasingly present today's physicians with a range of minor disorders that previous generations would not have even considered illness, and that we expect cures where no cures are possible. Michael Ignatieff, "Modern Dying," The New Republic, December 26, 1988, decries the overmedicalization of human sorrows, contending that "the more we define depression, sorrow, and pain as treatable conditions, the more insatiable we become for cures, the less reconciled we are to the instances when doctors cannot help us." (p. 31).

414. B. Belch, "Don't Blame The Victim," Newsweek, 1985.

415. Pascal James Imperato and Greg Mitchell, Acceptable Risks, New York: Viking, 1985, p. xix.

416. Robert L. Taylor, "Beware of Health Hype, "Reader's Digest, March, 1991, pp. 141-144. Condensed from his book: Health Fact, Health Fiction, Dallas, Texas: Taylor Publishing Company, 1990.

417. Stephen P. Maran, "Science Is Dandiny, But Promotion Can Be Lucrative," Smithsonian Magazine, May, 1991, pp. 72-80.

418. George Will, "Grandmother Was Right," Newsweek, January 16, 1989.

419. Michael Ignatieff, "Modern Dying," The New Republic, December 26, 1989, pp. 28-33.

420. George F. Will, 1989.

Notes to Chapter 16

421. Admittedly, the print is often so small that it can only be read with eyeglasses or a magnifying glass. This is especially frustrating for older persons.

422. Peggy Eastman, "Unlike 'Birds of a Feather,' Some Drugs Don't Go Together," AARP Bulletin, Vol. 30, No. 3, March, 1989.

423. Jane E. Brody, "Ignoring The Doctor's Orders Has Become a Costly and Deadly Epidemic," The New York Times, 1993.

424. Brody, Ibid.

425. Interestingly, physicians who become ill often exhibit lower compliance levels than patients.

426. J. Cameron, "A Few Irresistible Reasons for Paying Attention," Vogue, Vol. 171, 1981, p. 138.

427. Abigail J. Moss, et al, "Recent Trends in Adolescent Smoking, Smoking-Uptake Correlates, and Expectations About the Future," Advance Data From Vital and Health Statistics, No. 221, Hyattsville, Maryland: National Center for Health Statistics, December 2, 1992.

428. Fred Cutter, Coming to Terms With Death, Chicago: Nelson-Hall, 1974, p. 84.

429. "A Room and a Coffee Pot," <u>Royal Bank Letter</u>, Vol. 74, No. 3, May/June, 1993, pp. 1-4.

430. Timothy Elliot, "Negotiating Reality After Physical Loss: Hope, Depression, and Disability," <u>Journal of Personality and Social Psychology</u>, Vol. 61, No. 4., October, 1991, pp. 608-613.

431. Norman Cousins, <u>Head First: The Biology of Hope</u>, New York: E.P. Dutton, 1989.

432. Lionel Tiger, <u>Optimism: The Biology of Hope</u>, New York: Simon and Schuster, 1979, p. 40.

433. Martin E.P. Seligman, <u>Learned Optimism</u>, New York: Alfred A. Knopf, 1991.

434. Martin E.P. Seligman, "It Pays To Be An Optimist," <u>Bottom Line</u>, Vol. 12, No. 10, May 30, 1991, pp. 1-3.

435. "Miracle Drugs or Media Drugs?" <u>Consumer Reports</u>, March, 1992, pp. 142-146.

436. <u>Consumer Reports</u> March, 1992, pp. 145-46.

437. Earl Ubell, "Could You Use More Sleep?" <u>Parade Magazine</u>, January 10, 1993, pp. 20, 22, 24.

438. American Thoracic Society International Conference, San Diego, May 19-24, 2006.

439. Ibid.

440. An interesting contrast is the roughly 300,000 Americans who experience *narcolepsy*. They fall asleep without warning at any time, anywhere—obviously a potentially dangerous condition.

441. Damon Darlin, "Vet Bills and the Priceless Pet: What's a practical Owner to Do? The New York Times, May13, 2006, p. B1 and B6.

442. Sarah Burke, "In The Presence Of Animals," <u>U.S. News & World Report</u>, February 24, 1992, pp. 64-65.

443. Sarah Burke, 1992, p. 64.

444. Ibid, p. 65.

445. "Can You Live Longer?" <u>Consumer Reports</u>, January, 1992, pp. 1-15.

446. *Population Today.* The reader needs to keep in mind the demographic distinction between the concepts of *life span*—the theoretical biological limit for the species, the greatest age that a person living under ideal conditions would be able to reach, and *life expectancy*—the average age that a person in a given time and place, such as 20th century America, can expect to reach. To extend the human life span, it would be necessary to slow down the aging process. At the moment, there is no evidence that the human life span can be modified by any means. See: S. Jay Olshansky, "Estimating the Upper Limits to Human Longevity,", Vol. 20, No. 1, January, 1992, pp. 6-8.

447. John W. Travis and Regina Sara Ryan, "Wellness: Small Changes Can Make A Difference," <u>Bottom Line</u>, September 15, 1992, pp. 13-14.

448. "The Power of Little Things," <u>Royal Bank Newsletter</u>, Published by the Royal Bank of Canada, Vol. 74, No. 2, March\April, 1993.

449. Richard Conniff, "Living Longer," <u>Review Magazine</u>, August, 1981, pp. 62-65.

Notes to Chapter 17

450. Sheldon Krimsky and Dominic Golding, <u>Social Theories of Risk</u>, Westport, CT: Praeger, 1992.

451. Bob Davis, "What Price Safety? Risk Analysis Measures Need for Regulation, But It's No Science," <u>The Wall Street Journal</u>, August 6, 1992, pp. A1 & A4.

452. Gio Bata Gori, "Overturning the Verdict on Carcinogens," <u>Wall Street Journal</u>, August 27, 1992.

453. Michael R. Edelstein, <u>Contaminated Communities</u>, Boulder, CO: Westview Press, 1988, p. 142.

454. Edelstein, 1998, p. 145.

455. Phil Brown and Edwin J. Mikkelsen, <u>No Safe Place: Toxic Waste, Leukemia, and Community Action</u>, University of California Press, 1990.

456. Ibid. p. 126.

457. Examples of government, corporate, professional, or scientific resistance to citizen\community efforts to focus attention on environmental degradation sites, including getting those responsible to acknowledge their culpability, and to assume a restorative program, along with providing political, social, and economic redress, may be found in Brown and Mikkelsen (1990)

458. Brown and Mikkelsen, 1990, p. 131.

459. Brown and Mikkelsen (1990) argue that toxic waste activists apparently are generally dissatisfied with the new field of risk assessment because it "fails to take into account deeper social and cultural forces. The positivist cost-benefit analysis and psychometric studies of risk assessment cannot provide adequate information on health risks, because both the risks and perception of the risks are shaped by economic, ideological, and political concerns. Indeed, the very language of risk is highly subjective and controversial, laden with underlying political theories of society" (p. 152).

460. Donald B. Ardell, "The History and Future of Wellness," <u>Wellness Perspectives: Journal of Individual, Family, and Community Wellness</u>, Vol. 1, No. 1, Winter, 1984, pp. 3-23.

461. Robert Barnett, "Becoming A Type "H"—For Health," The Pfizer Healthcare Series, in <u>U.S. News & World Report</u>, 1991, p. A12.

462. Roger Walsh, <u>Staying Alive: The Psychology of Human Survival</u>, New Science Library\Shambhala Publications, 1985.

463. Robert McGarvey, "Traveling In The Comfort Zone," <u>USAir Magazine</u>, December, 1991, pp. 14-19.

464. Bobbie Sommer, psychotherapist, quoted in McGarvey, 1991, p. 18.

465. Experts in this area suggest several ways to avoid this in attempting to make lifestyle changes. One technique, sometimes called the building-block

approach, is to take small, more easily attainable steps first. Success and growing confidence then will lead you to take bigger, more challenging steps to alter your lifestyle. A related technique is to break large projects or goals down into a series of smaller steps. Then the task doesn't appear to overwhelming.

466. "Living With Uncertainty," <u>The Royal Bank Newsletter</u>, Vol. 68, No. 2, March/April, 1987.

467. Ibid, p. 4.

468. Ibid, p. 4.

978-0-595-40274-8
0-595-40274-7

www.ingramcontent.com/pod-product-compliance
Lightning Source LLC
Chambersburg PA
CBHW030259290526
45785CB00001B/146